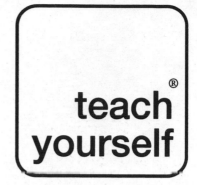

detox

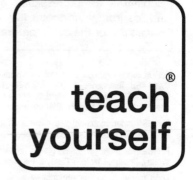

detox
denise whichello brown

The information written in this book is not intended as a substitute for professional advice. Always seek medical advice from your doctor if you are in any doubt as to your suitability for the detox programme.

For UK order enquiries: please contact Bookpoint Ltd, 130 Milton Park, Abingdon, Oxon, OX14 4SB. Telephone: +44 (0) 1235 827720. Fax: +44 (0) 1235 400454. Lines are open 09.00–17.00, Monday to Saturday, with a 24-hour message answering service. Details about our titles and how to order are available at www.teachyourself.co.uk

For USA order enquiries: please contact McGraw-Hill Customer Services, PO Box 545, Blacklick, OH 43004-0545, USA. Telephone: 1-800-722-4726. Fax: 1-614-755-5645.

For Canada order enquiries: please contact McGraw-Hill Ryerson Ltd, 300 Water St, Whitby, Ontario, L1N 9B6, Canada. Telephone: 905 430 5000. Fax: 905 430 5020.

Long renowned as the authoritative source for self-guided learning – with more than 50 million copies sold worldwide – the **teach yourself** series includes over 500 titles in the fields of languages, crafts, hobbies, business, computing and education.

British Library Cataloguing in Publication Data: a catalogue record for this title is available from the British Library.

Library of Congress Catalog Card Number: on file.

First published in UK 2004 by Hodder Education part of Hachette Livre UK, 338 Euston Road, London, NW1 3BH.

First published in US 2004 by The McGraw-Hill Companies, Inc.

This edition published 2004.

The **teach yourself** name is a registered trade mark of Hodder Headline.

Copyright © 2004 Denise Whichello Brown

Typeset by Transet Limited, Coventry, England.
Printed in Great Britain for Hodder Education, part of Hachette Livre UK, 338 Euston Road, London, NW1 3BH, by Cox & Wyman Ltd, Reading, Berkshire.

The publisher has used its best endeavours to ensure that the URLs for external websites referred to in this book are correct and active at the time of going to press. However, the publisher and the author have no responsibility for the websites and can make no guarantee that a site will remain live or that the content will remain relevant, decent or appropriate.

Hachette Livre UK's policy is to use papers that are natural, renewable and recyclable products and made from wood grown in sustainable forests. The logging and manufacturing processes are expected to conform to the environmental regulations of the country of origin.

Impression number   10 9 8 7 6
Year   2010 2009 2008 2007

contents

acknowledgements

For dearest Garry who types up all my work (how does he read my writing?).

For my beloved son, Tom, who hopes himself to be a famous writer someday.

For my beloved daughter, Chloe, who nags me if I don't have my five portions of fruit or vegetables per day and brings me lots of glasses of water. I must point out that though she knows everything about nutrition she conveniently forgets that chocolate is not on the detox list!

introduction

This easy-to-follow detox guide tells you all you need to know about how to look great and feel absolutely wonderful. It is *the* plan that will help you to totally transform your life. You will be amazed at the difference!

Everyone can benefit from a detox and if you choose to go down this road then you will discover the new re-energized, healthier and happier you!

Most detox books focus purely on physical detoxification and, of course, eating the right foods is absolutely vital – after all we are what we eat. However, it is not only physical toxins we need to clear. Cleansing the mind and spirit of toxins is also essential. In this comprehensive detox guide you will find all the tools to transform and energize all aspects of your life.

Prepare yourself for change and to look and feel younger and healthier in body, mind and spirit! What are you waiting for?

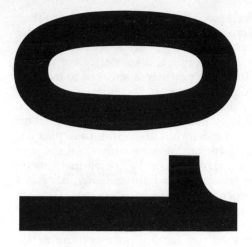

01

why detox?

In this chapter you will learn:
- about the reasons for detoxing
- whether you need a body detox
- about toxins and where they come from.

The majority of individuals pay a great deal of attention to their outward physical appearance. They bath or shower on a regular basis, shampoo and condition their hair frequently and religiously brush their teeth. Creams and cosmetics are applied to enhance the way we look and perfume is spritzed to make us smell attractive. Cosmetic surgery too is becoming increasingly popular to smooth away the years. All this attention is devoted to the outside of our bodies but what about the inside? Our inner cleanliness is vital and indeed has an enormous impact not only on the way that we look but also, of course, on the way that we feel. Many individuals are becoming increasingly aware of the importance of detoxification and are realizing that it's a powerful tool not only to enhance our physical appearance but also for the prevention of disease and the maintenance of optimum health. Everyone can benefit from the process of detoxification and if we used this natural process more in our daily lives many illnesses could be prevented and healed.

Reasons to detox

All of us are toxic to a certain degree – some of us more so than others! If you are suffering from any of the following complaints then it is time for a detox for all of these symptoms are warning signs of possible health problems later on in life.

- Poor energy levels
- Sluggish metabolism and an inability to lose weight
- Skin problems
- Dull hair
- Poor nails
- Tired eyes
- Bowel problems
- Digestive disorders
- Bloatedness
- Headaches
- Aches and pains
- Bad breath
- Coated tongue
- Mouth ulcers
- Cracked/Chapped lips
- Fluid retention
- Menstrual problems
- Insomnia
- Excessive worrying
- Anger and irritability
- Mood swings
- Cellulite
- Allergies
- High cholesterol
- Blocked arteries
- Stress and tension
- Depression
- Inability to concentrate
- Drowsiness
- Woolly head feeling
- Memory loss
- Inability to focus
- Difficulty with creativity and making changes.

Toxins are a major cause of ill health and if you just give your body the chance to throw off these poisons then you can achieve optimum health. Instead of reaching for painkillers for headaches and aches and pains, antacids for indigestion, laxatives for constipation, caffeine for tiredness, cigarettes and alcohol for relaxation and sleeping tablets for insomnia and so on, why not give detoxification a try? Need more convincing? Then try out the following questionnaire!

Questionnaire – do you need a body detox?

Find out how healthy you are and discover whether your body is crying out for a spring clean.

1   How good is your diet?
    Very healthy   2
    Fairly balanced   1
    Unhealthy   0

2   Do you skip breakfast?
    Never   2
    Sometimes   1
    Always   0

3   Do you eat sugary snacks (i.e. sweets, biscuits, cakes) between meals?
    Never   2
    Sometimes   1
    Always   0

4   Do you eat salted snacks (i.e. crisps) between meals?
    Never   2
    Sometimes   1
    Every day   0

5   How many fresh portions of fruit and vegetables do you eat daily?
    5+   2
    2–4   1
    0–1   0

6   How much water do you drink daily?
    6–8 glasses   2
    A couple of glasses   1
    None   0

7 How many units of alcohol do you drink per week?
0–4	2
5–8	1
More than 8	0

8 How many cups of coffee or tea do you drink daily?
None	2
Less than 6	1
More than 6	0

9 Do you drink fizzy and soft drinks?
Never	2
Sometimes	1
Often	0

10 How many cigarettes do you smoke daily?
None	2
5 or less	1
5+	0

11 How often do you have takeaways/fast food?
Never	2
Once a week	1
Often	0

12 Do you eat ready meals?
Never	2
At least once a week	1
Often	0

13 Do you eat when you're not hungry or when you are bored or stressed?
Never	2
Sometimes	1
Often	0

14 Do you find yourself craving certain foods?
Never	2
Sometimes	1
Often	0

15 Do you often try to diet?
Never	2
Sometimes	1
I am constantly on a diet	0

16 Is it difficult to lose weight?
No 2
Fairly difficult 1
Yes, very difficult 0

17 Do you take over-the-counter medications such as asprin and paracetamol?
Never/Rarely 2
At least once a week 1
Often 0

18 Do you feel tired and lethargic?
Never 2
Occasionally 1
Most/All of the time 0

19 Do you often feel bloated?
Never 2
Sometimes 1
Often 0

20 Do you suffer with heartburn/indigestion/flatulence?
Never 2
Sometimes 1
Often 0

21 Do you suffer with irritable bowel syndrome?
Never 2
Sometimes 1
Often 0

22 Do you suffer with constipation?
No 2
Rarely 1
Sometimes 0

23 Do you have allergies?
None 2
One or two 1
Lots 0

24 Are you prone to skin problems?
Never 2
I get the odd spot or two 1
Often 0

25 Is your hair dry/dull/lacking in lustre?
Never 2
Sometimes 1
Often 0

26 Are your nails brittle and flaky?
Never 2
Sometimes 1
Often 0

27 Do you suffer with headaches?
Never 2
Sometimes 1
Often 0

28 Is your breath bad and is your tongue coated?
Never 2
Sometimes 1
Often 0

29 Do you suffer with menstrual irregularities such as premenstrual tension (PMT)?
Never 2
Sometimes 1
Often 0

30 Do you have cellulite?
No 2
Very slightly 1
Yes 0

31 Do you recover quickly from an illness such as a cold?
Yes 2
Within a week or two 1
It lingers on 0

32 Do your joints feel stiff and your muscles ache?
Never 2
Sometimes 1
Often 0

33 Do you suffer from fluid retention?
Never 2
Sometimes 1
Often 0

34 Do you sleep well?
Always 2
Usually 1
Hardly ever/Never 0

35 Are you prone to mood swings and irritability?
Never 2
Sometimes 1
Often 0

36 Do you find it difficult to focus and concentrate?
Never 2
Sometimes 1
Often 0

37 Do you feel depressed and tearful?
Never 2
Sometimes 1
Often 0

38 Is your memory sharp?
Always 2
Most of the time 1
Not often/Never 0

39 Does your head feel 'woolly'?
Never 2
Sometimes 1
Often 0

40 Do you find it difficult to motivate yourself?
Never 2
Sometimes 1
Often 0

Your answers

How did you do?

60+

If your score is over 60 you seem to be in good health. However, by following my detox plan you should be able to feel even more energetic and positively glow with health!

31–60

If your score is between 31 and 60 then it seems that your body is out of balance. Although you do not feel 'ill' there are some warning signs that all is not as it should be. Now is the time to heed those alarm bells and to detox before your symptoms get any worse! Keep all those vital organs of elimination working to their full capacity and rid yourself of those toxins.

0–30

If your score is between 0 and 30 then you certainly need to detox! You seem to be suffering from a lot of health complaints which could be caused by your poor eating habits and your body is likely to be overburdened with junk food. Your body is longing for a cleanse and some healthy nutrients.

What are toxins and where do they come from?

A toxin can be defined as any poisonous substance which is detrimental to the optimum functioning of the body and thus our health and well-being. Toxins are responsible for creating harmful and irritating effects in our bodies thus disturbing the homeostasis – equilibrium or balance of the body.

Toxicity is a far bigger problem in the 21st century than ever before. In days gone by the majority of individuals did not have to deal with the thousands of toxic chemicals to which we are now unfortunately exposed to on a daily basis. Toxic substances include poor diet, caffeine, alcohol, cigarettes, drugs, heavy metals, chemicals, radiation, pollution and even stress and tension.

Dietary toxins

An average diet is not necessarily a healthy one for we eat and drink toxins regularly and repeatedly. In the 21st century toxicity is of greater concern than ever before since we interfere far too much with our natural foods. In order to improve yields farmers add chemicals such as herbicides, pesticides, insecticides and artificial fertilizers. Any crops that are not organically grown are universally grown with nitrate fertilizers, and pesticides and herbicides are sprayed on vegetables, fruits, grains and so on. Even when the crops have been harvested they are still not safe from chemicals – for instance, potatoes, whilst in store, are treated with anti-sprouting chemicals, and gases are used to artificially ripen fruit. These residues find their way onto our plates and adversely influence our bodies. Indeed they have been implicated in cancer, liver damage, infertility, allergic diseases and a whole host of other problems.

Farmers regularly feed or inject their animals with chemicals and hormones to promote growth and add antibiotics to their feed. Not only the meat but also our eggs and dairy produce will be laced with these chemicals. Even small quantities of these drugs are thought to cause disruption of our intestinal bacteria increasing the likelihood of allergies and yeast and fungus growth.

The food industry adds thousands of unnecessary substances to our food such as preservatives, stabilizers, taste enhancers, artificial colourings and flavourings, which are all detrimental to our health. These substances are added to food to reduce its rate of deterioration to create a longer shelf life and to make foods more appealing. These contaminated foods often cause allergic reactions in sensitive individuals, interfere with digestion and put stress on our immune systems.

Some particularly troublesome additives include the yellow colouring tartrazine (E102) which can cause allergic reactions, the nitrates (E249–52) which are preservatives used in curing meats and have been associated with cancer. The antioxidant gallates (E310–12) can induce gastric irritation and monosodium glutamate, a flavour enhancer, also causes adverse effects.

Fresh foods (preferably organic), free from additives and preservatives are essential for our health and well-being.

Drugs

Many modern drugs are lifesaving but they can interact with nutrients and affect the absorption of our nutrients. The wide range of over-the-counter drugs and prescribed medication that the majority of people rely on can have side effects and if taken in excess can lead to hospitalization. Addiction to over-the-counter drugs is increasingly becoming a problem. I am not suggesting, of course, that anyone should stop taking any medication(s) prescribed by the doctor but sometimes it is possible to treat the cause of an illness with detoxification and a new nutritional regime.

Did you know that:

- Drugs adversely affect the liver and damage brain cells.
- Aspirins may reduce vitamin C levels.
- Diuretics cause an increase in loss of magnesium, zinc and potassium.
- Antibiotics (especially long-term courses) interfere with the balance of intestinal flora allowing yeasts and moulds to flourish.
- Oestrogen based oral contraceptives have a detrimental effect on the B vitamins, zinc and folic acid.
- Antacids contain aluminium which has been implicated in Alzheimer's disease.
- Tranquillizers deplete many nutrients especially vitamins C and B.
- Corticosteroids lower zinc levels.

Therefore, drugs should be avoided unless they are absolutely necessary!

Alcohol

Alcohol, if drunk in moderation, will not cause any harm but if it is misused it can damage the body. The minerals and vitamins which are depleted include the vitamins B and C, folic acid, calcium, magnesium, potassium, zinc as well as the essential fatty acids.

Long-term consumption of excessive alcohol damages the liver, brain and nervous system, heart, oesophagus, pancreas and stomach. The risk of gout is increased, fat levels in the blood are raised and diabetes is worsened. If alcohol is drunk during pregnancy this can lead to mental retardation of the child.

Caffeine

Caffeine is a very powerful drug that is present in tea, coffee, cola and even chocolate. An average cup of strong tea contains 50 mg of caffeine and a cup of coffee contains 100 mg. Any dose exceeding 250 mg can produce significant pharmacological effects. According to the *British Medical Journal*, individuals who drink five cups of coffee daily have a 50 per cent greater chance of having a heart attack. Coffee has been shown to raise levels of bad cholesterol and blood fats and can damage the liver. Caffeine can also result in excessive urination and diarrhoea and reduces iron absorption if consumed at mealtimes. It acts directly on the nervous system and too much will induce nervousness, depression and insomnia.

Interestingly, decaffeinated drinks do not provide a solution as although the caffeine has been removed the chemicals theophylline and theobromine remain. These chemicals affect humans in a similar way to caffeine!

Smoking

Cigarette smoke contains 2,000 chemicals including nicotine, tar, arsenic, cyanide and cadmium. Not a healthy concoction! Smoking causes damage to the circulatory system, affecting the heart and lungs. It can elevate blood pressure and damage the liver. Smoking also affects digestion and has an adverse effect on vitamin C levels. Just one cigarette can increase vitamin C requirements by 25 mg.

If you smoke, a detox will curb your need for cigarettes.

Environmental pollution and toxic metals

We live in a very toxic environment and it is impossible to avoid pollution. Toxins can be acquired by breathing them in, by ingesting them or by direct physical contact. It is not only outdoor pollution and traffic fumes and poisoned industrial processes that we need to concern ourselves with but also indoor pollution. We are exposed to chemicals from cleaning materials, fumes from our gas appliances and electromagnetic fields from computers, mobile phones, televisions and electric clock radios.

We are also exposed to toxic metals such as lead, aluminium, mercury and cadmium. Such substances are also known as antinutrients since they compromise our nutritional status by interfering with our uptake of essential nutrients.

Lead

Toxicity can arise from:

- Atmospheric lead – e.g. traffic pollution and industry
- Lead water pipes and drinking water
- Leaded house paint
- Cigarettes
- Lead toys and pencils
- Hair dyes.

The adverse effects of lead include:

- Nervous system problems
- Hyperactivity in children, behavioural disorders and impaired IQ
- Cancer
- Cardiovascular disease such as high blood pressure and hardening of the arteries
- Poor immune function.

Aluminium

Sources of aluminium toxicity include:

- Cookware, household and industrial utensils
- Some table salts where aluminium salts have been added to prevent it from attracting water and becoming difficult to pour
- Aluminium foil
- Antiperspirants
- Antacids
- Bleached flour
- Toothpaste.

Overexposure to aluminium can result in:

- Problems with the central nervous system such as Alzheimer's disease (pre-senile dementia)
- Childhood hyperactivity

- Dyslexia
- Liver and kidney disorders.

Mercury

Mercury toxicity can arise from:

- Amalgam fillings – mercury vapour is released from fillings especially when one chews
- Fungicides and pesticides
- Fish.

The effects of mercury toxicity include:

- Mental and neurological symptoms possibly implicated in multiple sclerosis
- Chronic fatigue
- Suppression of the immune system
- Kidney and liver damage.

Cadmium

Sources of cadmium toxicity include:

- Cigarettes (16 to 24 mg per cigarette)
- Rubber tyres and plastics
- Red and yellow pigments
- Insecticides
- Refined and canned foods
- New carpets
- Detergents.

Effects of cadmium toxicity include:

- High blood pressure
- Kidney damage
- Nervous system problems
- Respiratory disorders.

Other toxic metals include copper (from water pipes), arsenic (found in some table salts, beers and wines, dyes, paints) and fluoride (present in toothpaste, fluoridated water and non-stick pans).

You should try to avoid exposure to these toxic metals both at home and work, eat seaweed and plenty of nutrient-rich fruit and vegetables and take a detoxifying vitamin C supplement.

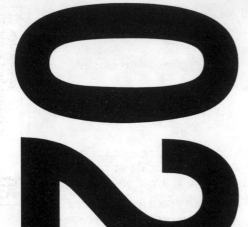

02

know your organs of elimination

In this chapter you will learn:
• about how your body eliminates toxins.

The body has natural methods of detoxification and toxins may be excreted via the liver, kidneys, colon, skin, lungs and lymphatic system.

Let us take a brief look at each of these organs and their eliminative functions:

The liver

Apart from the skin, the liver is the largest organ in the body. It weighs about 1.4 kg (about 3 lb) and is situated just beneath the diaphragm. The liver has remarkable powers of regeneration provided it has not been too badly damaged.

The liver performs many essential functions including the following:

Detoxification

The liver is a major organ of detoxification. Poisonous compounds such as alcohol, drugs and other substances enter the blood from the intestines and on reaching the liver are converted to harmless substances and later excreted. Also when amino acids that are not required for making protein are converted, toxic nitrogenous wastes such as ammonia are produced and are processed by the liver. This toxic waste is converted into urea by the liver, which is a fairly harmless substance that is eliminated via the kidneys (in our urine) and also by our sweat glands. Thus, the liver is vital for the removal of poisonous substances.

Production of bile

Liver cells secrete about a pint of bile a day which is made up of bile salts (formed in the liver from cholesterol), bile pigments and cholesterol. Bile salts are important for the emulsification (breakdown) and absorption of fats. The liver recycles 80 per cent of bile salts to once again become part of the bile. Bile is a green colour due to the pigments bilirubin (red) and biliverdin (green), which are derived from haemoglobin.

Since the liver plays an important part in the breakdown of fats, the health of our liver is a consideration if we are to avoid diseases such as blocked arteries and obesity.

Storage

The liver stores the fat soluble vitamins A, D, E and K, vitamin B12 and also the mineral iron. The liver also stores poisons that cannot be broken down such as DDT which can be found in the livers of humans and animals who eat fruits and vegetables that have been sprayed. A good reason to eat organic fruit and vegetables.

Synthesises vitamin A

The liver synthesises vitamin A from carotene that is found in abundance in green leafy vegetables and carrots.

Plasma proteins

The liver produces most of the proteins (from amino acids) found in blood plasma such as albumin, globulin, prothrombin and fibrinogen which play an important part in blood clotting. The clotting of blood is essential not only to stop further blood loss but also to prevent the entry of harmful bacteria into cuts and wounds.

Production of heat

The liver is the primary heat-producing organ of the body as a result of all its functions. If your liver is working too hard you will feel hot whereas if your liver is sluggish then you can experience low energy levels.

Regulation of blood sugar

After we have eaten a meal the liver removes any excess glucose (sugar) from the blood and stores it as glycogen. In between meals when the concentration of glucose in the blood starts to fall the liver converts some of the stored glycogen into glucose and releases the glucose into the bloodstream. This maintains our blood sugar at a constant level.

If we eat too much sugar and refined carbohydrates such as cakes, biscuits, white bread and white rice then our blood sugar levels go haywire so that we experience highs and lows of energy levels and excess blood glucose is turned into unwanted fat.

The kidneys

The kidneys play a key role in detoxification. They cleanse the blood of toxic substances such as urea and other nitrogenous (i.e. waste products containing nitrogen) waste. The kidneys also expel excess water, salts and hormones. These waste products are excreted by the kidneys in our urine. On average every 24 hours about 1.5 litres of urine is produced. However, urine output may be increased by our liquid intake or cold weather and decreased by factors such as high temperatures and exercise which increase sweating.

To ensure that our kidneys are removing waste products effectively we need to try to drink 2 litres of water per day. A diet that is rich in fruits and vegetables which have a high water content is also advisable.

You can tell if you need more water by the colour of your urine. If your urine is cloudy or dark or has an unpleasant aroma then you need to increase your fluid intake. Tiredness, lethargy, headaches, nausea, poor concentration and dry skin are just a few of the other symptoms of dehydration (for more information see page 74). If the kidneys are put under too much pressure then more serious problems such as kidney infections or even kidney stones may arise.

The colon

One of the primary functions of the colon (large intestine) is to excrete our waste. This waste material consists of water, undigested food, cellulose and vegetable fibres (roughage), dead blood cells, mucus and bacteria. You may be surprised to learn that the normal colon contains 1.4–1.8 kg of bacteria! One of the functions of these beneficial bacteria is to control infection from harmful yeasts, fungi, bacteria, viruses and worms.

We could learn a great deal from observing our faeces. They should be quite bulky, soft and a mid-brown colour and they should be easily passed. Motions should not be sticky or smelly and we should empty our bowels at least once a day and preferably two or three times. Stools that look like rabbit droppings are not indicative of a healthy colon! A good detox followed by a healthy eating programme will help to eliminate symptoms such as constipation, diarrhoea and excess gas.

The skin

The skin is the largest organ in the body with an area of 1.6–1.9 m^2 in an average adult. It has a wide range of functions including protection, temperature regulation, sensations, synthesis of vitamin D, secretion and of course elimination.

Toxins are eliminated via the sweat glands. On an average day approximately half a litre of sweat is lost and a great deal more on a hot day or if we are physically active. Waste products such as water and salts are eliminated via our sweat glands.

Our skin is an indication as to what is happening on the inside of the body. If you suffer with spots and blemishes then you need to detox. A healthy glowing complexion is one of the benefits of this programme.

The lungs

The respiratory system, of which the lungs are a major part, is an important system of elimination. It takes in substances from the environment and the oxygen is taken up by the blood whereas the waste and carbon dioxide are expelled.

Unfortunately, the air is full of pollution and we breathe in not only desirable oxygen but also traffic fumes, industrial and household chemicals, dust, moulds, cigarette smoke and so on.

The majority of us breathe in a very shallow manner and by learning to breathe deeply we can increase the elimination of toxins through our lungs (see page 121).

The lymphatic system

Your lymphatic system can be thought of as your body's waste disposal system. It is an extensive system distributed throughout the body that neutralizes and drains away excess tissue fluid, dead cells and harmful waste and toxins. The lymph carries the waste products to the organs of elimination. It also plays an important part in the body's immune and defence system. Lymph nodes filter the lymph, destroying harmful micro-organisms, thus preventing toxins from passing into the bloodstream. If the lymph is not flowing freely around the body, symptoms such as swelling, particularly around the ankles, behind the knees, and around the wrists, may be apparent. The

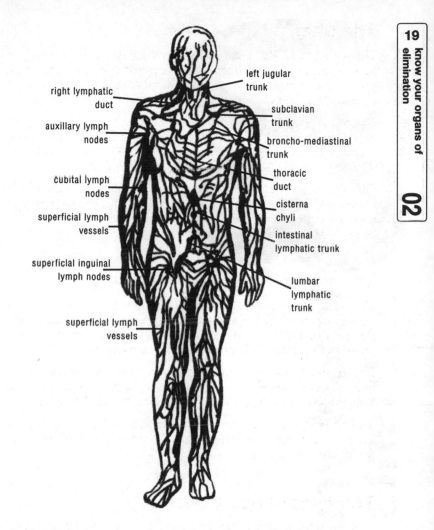

right lymphatic
duct

auxillary lymph
nodes

cubital lymph
nodes

superficial lymph
vessels

superficial inguinal
lymph nodes

superficial lymph
vessels

left jugular
trunk

subclavian
trunk

broncho-mediastinal
trunk

thoracic
duct

cisterna
chyli

intestinal
lymphatic trunk

lumbar
lymphatic
trunk

figure 1 the lymphatic system

lymphatic system can be cleansed by drinking 2 litres of water
daily and also by exercise since the contraction of skeletal
muscles directs the lymph around the body. Dry skin brushing
(see page 94) is also an excellent way of stimulating the
lymphatic system.

03

know your nutrients

In this chapter you will learn:
- about the vital nutrients required by the body to function at an optimum level
- about good sources of these nutrients
- what happens if you are deficient.

During a detox it is essential that the requirements of all the vital nutrients are met so that the body is able to function at its optimum level.

What are the vital nutrients?

The vital nutrients are:

- Amino acids (proteins)
- Carbohydrates
- Essential fatty acids (fats)
- Vitamins
- Minerals
- Dietary fibre
- Water
- Oxygen

and emotional nutrients such as love!

Amino acids (protein)

The word 'protein' is derived from the Greek and means 'of first importance'. It is essential for the formation of bone, connective tissue (skin), hair and muscle. Functional proteins include antibodies, digestive enzymes and hormones such as insulin. Proteins are composed of building blocks known as amino acids. Our bodies need 20 different amino acids, but we are able to make 12 of these from the following eight, which we must get from food: tryptophan, lysine, methionine, phenylalanine, threonine, valine, leucine and isoleucine.

It should be remembered that although protein is essential, too much is a common mistake in the Western diet. The body only requires approximately 50 gms of protein daily. If more protein is ingested than required then some of it may be incompletely digested with the poisonous by-products leading to arthritis, mucous, headaches, allergies and so on. Care should be taken when protein is eaten in the form of red meat.

Too much red meat has been linked with heart disease, strokes and cancer and meat remains in the colon for long periods putrefying and toxifying the colon. In addition, antibodies, chemicals and growth hormones are often added. Choose preferably lean organically reared meat in small quantities.

Too many dairy foods can cause the overproduction of mucous, allergies, arthritis, asthma, colds, migraines and so on. Try alternatives such as goat's milk, cheese and butter, feta cheese, mozzarella cheese and soya products. Fish is an excellent protein – oily fish such as mackerel is especially beneficial.

Pulses, seeds and nuts are also beneficial sources of protein.

Carbohydrates

The main function of carbohydrates is to provide energy. However, it is very important not to choose foods high in refined processed sugars. High sugar foods are popular but they are low in essential nutrients and are referred to as 'empty calories'. They give rise to obesity, cardiovascular disease, diabetes, gastrointestinal disease, tooth decay, depression and anxiety, mood swings, hyperactivity in children and skin problems. It is an alarming fact that in the UK approximately 40–50 kg of sugar are consumed per head each year (30 teaspoons per day)! Apart from the obvious sources such as biscuits, cakes, jams, puddings, sweets and fizzy drinks there is a considerable amount of 'hidden sugars' in our food. Tinned and packet foods are full of sugar.

Good sources of carbohydrate include grains (whole brown rice, whole wheat, barley, rye, oats), root vegetables (such as carrots), fruit (such as bananas) and pulses (such as lentils, peas and beans).

Fats

The basic building blocks of fats are fatty acids. They may be saturated or unsaturated. Saturated fatty acids are mainly present in hard fats such as butter, lard, animal fats and coconut and palm oils. They are solid at room temperature. Eating too much saturated fat has been linked with a high risk of heart disease and raised blood pressure and cholesterol levels as well as weight gain.

Unsaturated fatty acids are divided into two types – monounsaturated and polyunsaturated. Monounsaturates such as in olive oil, rapeseed oil and avocado pears are considered to be healthy. In Mediterranean countries, where enormous amounts of olive oil are consumed, the incidence of heart disease is low. To promote health, whenever possible use cold-pressed vegetable oils instead of saturated fats.

Polyunsaturates are also regarded as healthy. Polyunsaturated fatty acids are often called essential fatty acids (EFAs) and are present in seed and vegetable oils, nuts and seeds, oily fish and lean meat. EFAs are thought to prevent heart disease (Eskimos have a very low rate of cardiac disease) and may also benefit inflammatory conditions (e.g. eczema), PMT, multiple sclerosis and hyperactivity.

Vitamins

Vitamins are organic substances essential for life which must be obtained from food (if not from dietary supplements). If a healthy balanced diet is consumed then supplements should not be necessary. Excesses of supplements should never be taken as they can be dangerous. For instance, too much vitamin A is toxic and can cause liver damage. You cannot take vitamin pills, stop eating and expect to be healthy.

The main vitamins together with their functions, sources and the effect of deficiency are listed below:

Vitamin A

Functions:

- Healthy eye function
- Helps skin conditions – especially dry skin and acne
- Mucous membranes (lungs, nose, throat)
- Strengthens the immune system.

Deficiency:

- Night blindness.

Good food sources:

- Animal and fish livers
- Fish liver oils
- Carrots
- Green and yellow vegetables.

Vitamin B complex

The B vitamins work together as a team and they tend to occur in the same foods.

When using any individual B vitamin as a supplement, it should always be taken along with the full B complex to ensure a balance is maintained.

Functions:

- Vital for the functioning of the nervous system helping to alleviate irritation and depression
- Important for the storage and release of energy
- Maintains healthy skin.

Deficiency:

- Beriberi (B1)
- Ariboflavinosis – mouth, lips, skin (B2)
- Pellagra – dermatitis, diarrhoea, dementia (B3)
- Seborrheic dermatitis, in severe cases anaemia (B6)
- Pernicious anaemia (B12) – injections are given for pernicious anaemia.

Good food sources:

- Brewer's yeast
- Fortified cereals
- Wholegrains
- Dairy foods
- Meat.

Folic acid

Functions:

- Essential for early pregnancy
- Vital for the formation of red blood cells.

Deficiency:

- Risk of spina bifida (folic acid has a protective effect against neural tube defects)
- Anaemia.

Good food sources:

- Green leafy vegetables (raw)
- Avocado
- Offal

- Wholegrain cereals
- Bananas.

Vitamin C

Functions:

- Essential for the formation of connective tissue (which forms all bones, cartilage, tendons, ligaments, dermis of the skin, etc.)
- Promotes healing
- Boosts the immune system
- Detoxifying
- Aids the absorption of iron.

Deficiency:

- Scurvy (severe deficiency)
- Bleeding gums, delayed wound healing, frequent infections.

Good food sources:

- Fresh fruit – especially blackcurrants, rosehips, strawberries, citrus and tropical fruits
- Raw peppers
- Green leafy vegetables
- Tomatoes
- Potatoes.

Vitamin D

Functions:

- Vital for the health of teeth and bones
- Essential for the absorption of calcium.

Deficiency:

- Rickets in children – bow-shaped legs, knock knees and pigeon-chests
- Osteomalacia in adults – softening of the bones causing fractures.

Good sources:

- Sunlight
- Oily fish – sardines, herring. mackerel, tuna
- Dairy products.

Vitamin E

Functions:

- Protects against heart disease and cancer
- Acts as an antioxidant keeping you looking younger
- Accelerates the healing of scars and burns
- Useful for infertility, menstrual and menopausal disorders.

Deficiency:

- Some types of anaemia
- Reproductive disorders.

Good food sources:

- Seed oils and vegetable oils
- Green vegetables
- Wholegrains
- Egg yolks.

Vitamin K

Functions:

- Essential for normal blood clotting – it is known as the anti-haemorrhage vitamin.

Deficiency:

- Excessive bleeding
- Haemorrhages in babies (newborn babies are given vitamin K injections).

Good food sources

- Green leafy vegetables
- Egg yolks
- Live yoghurt
- Kelp
- Alfalfa
- Vegetable and fish liver oils.

Minerals

Minerals are inorganic substances that perform a wide range of functions throughout the body. Some of the principal minerals are as follows:

Calcium

Functions:

- Vital for strong and healthy bones and teeth
- Essential for normal nerve function – it is calming and aids sleep
- Important for muscle function.

Deficiency:

- Osteoporosis (brittle bones)
- Osteomalacia (adults) and rickets (children)
- Cramps and convulsions
- Nervousness.

Good food sources:

- Dairy products
- Sardines
- Green vegetables
- Sesame seeds
- Sunflower and pumpkin seeds.

Iron

Functions:

- Essential for the formation of haemoglobin
- Maximizes energy
- Promotes resistance to disease.

The body's need for iron increases during menstruation and pregnancy.

Deficiency:

- Anaemia.

Good food sources (NB vitamin C is essential for iron absorption):

- Liver, kidneys and heart
- Meat
- Egg yolk
- Shellfish
- Molasses
- Lentils
- Nuts
- Wholegrains.

Magnesium

Functions:

- Essential for healthy nerves and muscles
- As a natural tranquillizer it reduces stress
- Helps to maintain brain functions.

Deficiency:

- Poor calcium deposition
- Cramps, muscle twitches and tremors
- Irritability
- Insomnia
- Hyperactivity in children.

Good food sources:

- Green leafy vegetables
- Wholegrains
- Nuts
- Seeds
- Bananas
- Avocados.

Phosphorus

Functions:

- Vital for the building and maintenance of bones and teeth
- Speeds up bone healing
- Provides energy.

Deficiency:

- Rickets (children) and osteomalacia (adults)
- Fatigue.

Good food sources (phosphorus is widely distributed):

- Dairy products
- Meat
- Fish
- Nuts and seeds
- Brewer's yeast
- Wholegrains.

Potassium

Functions:

- It works with sodium to regulate the body's water balance and regulate heart rhythms
- Vital for nerve function.

Deficiency:

- Muscle weakness
- Oedema
- Apathy

Good food sources:

- Avocados
- Bananas
- Lentils
- Dried and fresh fruits
- Meat
- Poultry.

Zinc

Functions:

- Vital for growth
- Essential for the nervous system
- Speeds healing of wounds
- Boosts the immune system
- Prevents stretch marks and prostrate problems.

Deficiency:

- Lack of growth
- Reproductive disorders
- Increased infections

- Loss of taste and smell
- Delayed wound healing.

Good food sources:

- Red meat
- Liver
- Shellfish
- Eggs
- Wholegrains
- Pulses.

Dietary fibre (roughage)

A diet which is high in fibre is often a healthy nutrient-dense diet in contrast to a diet low in fibre which is unhealthy and high in fat and sugar.

Fibre is present in all plant foods including cereals and vegetables, pulses, fruits, nuts and seeds. Dietary fibre is helpful for alleviating constipation and diverticular disease. High-fibre diets are associated with a lower incidence of cancer of the colon. A high-fibre diet also appears to protect against coronary heart disease although more research is needed. Diabetics are advised to eat a diet high in fibre as it reduces the swings in blood sugar levels that follow meals which contain high quantities of simple sugars.

Water

Water constitutes about two thirds of the body's weight. A human being can live for weeks without food, but only a few days without water. Under ordinary circumstances at least six to eight glasses of water daily is considered to be healthy.

Water is necessary to keep all our bodily functions working. It is essential for removing waste, helps to prevent constipation and regulates body temperature.

04

preparation for your detox

In this chapter you will learn:
- how to prepare yourself before a detox
- about the best time to detox
- possible side effects of detoxing
- about the benefits of the detox
- about the items you will need for the detox.

Before your detox

Caution! You should not follow any detoxification programme without seeking medical advice if any of the following applies to you:

- you are pregnant
- you are breastfeeding
- you are currently undergoing any medical treatment for any physical or mental illness
- you are taking any medications
- you are recovering from a serious illness
- you have just undergone any major surgery, as the body has weakened and needs all its energy for healing
- you are suffering from an eating disorder
- you are a growing child.

If you are in any doubt whatsoever about your suitability to detox, seek advice from a medically-qualified practitioner.

The best time to detox

It is a good idea to plan your detox in advance and look upon it in a very positive way. Look forward to the improvements that you're going to make to your current state of health and well-being. You can really make a powerful impact on your life.

You can begin at any time of the year, although a particularly appropriate time is in the early part of the year after you have recovered from your Christmas and New Year festivities. You may well have overindulged and your body will be crying out for a cleanse!

Try to pick a time when you do not have too many social commitments or distractions so that it is easier to keep focused on your detox regime. Do not try to begin a few days before your birthday, the week before your child's birthday party, or when you are due to go away for business, necessitating staying in a hotel. At these times, you will find yourself surrounded by all sorts of unsuitable foods as well as coffee and alcohol. You may not be able to resist, and even if you can, your friends and colleagues may not be very sympathetic towards your eating plan!

There is absolutely no need to take time off work, as the detox regime should fit easily into your lifestyle. It is a good idea to begin at the weekend when you have a couple of days at home so that you can plan your recipes for the week and rest, if you need to. In your first week try not to arrange too many social engagements and if you are eating with friends try to entertain them in your own home. They will not even be aware that they are on the detox as there is a whole host of exciting recipes in this book to choose from.

Try not to look upon the detox programme as a chore. You should look forward to it for you will be trying out lots of new foods, pampering yourself and discovering a new you that is full of energy and vitality. Enjoy!

Possible side effects

My detox programme is designed to involve the minimum amount of side effects with the maximum amount of health benefits. It is a gentle detox but do not be alarmed if you experience any of the following symptoms. They are all common reactions, which will pass away fairly quickly. Any of these reactions should be looked on in a positive light for they are signs that your body (and mind) are successfully eliminating toxins.

Fatigue
Do not be too surprised if you feel tired for the first few days as your organs of elimination will be working overtime. Soon you will begin to feel much more energetic.

Constipation
Any change in dietary habits can result in constipation. Often when we go on a holiday we find that it takes our bowels a while to adjust. Make sure that you are drinking plenty of water and, if necessary, increase your fruit and vegetable intake. Try not to use a laxative. Simply drink a glass of fruit juice or eat a few prunes and figs.

Loose bowels
You may find that your bowel movements become loose due to an increased intake of fibre.

Increase in the frequency and bulk of stools
It could happen that you have to make frequent visits to the loo. Your bowel movements could increase to three times a day. This is an excellent sign indicating that the detox is working and your bowels are working effectively.

Headaches

If you have been drinking lots of tea, coffee or caffeinated soft drinks you could have withdrawal symptoms and therefore experience mild headaches lasting for up to three days. Make sure that you are drinking your 2 litres of water daily to help to avoid or at least minimize this reaction.

Coated tongue

A fuzzy or coated tongue is commonly experienced during a detox. You may even have a nasty taste in your mouth or think that your breath is smelly. Again this is a sign that your body is eliminating toxins. To counteract this you can invest in a tongue scraper or brush your tongue with your toothbrush to make it fresh and clean. Alternatively you can rinse your mouth out with the juice of half a lemon squeezed in half a glass of water.

Increase in perspiration

As we have seen, the skin is an organ of elimination. If more toxins than usual are being eliminated via your sweat glands you may find that you're a little smelly to begin with. A good excuse for a wonderful aromatherapy shower or bath!

Spots and pimples

As your skin is ridding itself of waste matter you may find that initially the odd spot will appear. This is perfectly normal and soon your complexion will clear and take on a glowing healthy appearance.

Changes in urination

Your urine can become cloudy and unpleasant and increase in frequency. If this occurs then increase your water intake to encourage your kidneys to eliminate the waste products. Be aware that vitamin supplements can change the colour of your urine often to a bright yellow colour. Freshly-juiced fruit and vegetables can also produce colour changes. Have you ever noticed that beetroot turns the urine pink?

Nasal discharges

If you have a problem with catarrh it is possible that for a few days you will experience a nasal discharge or even a mild cough as your body takes advantage of the opportunity to rid itself of mucus.

Anger/Irritability

You may be surprised that a detox can induce emotional changes too. As you detox your body you will also be detoxing your mind and your spirit too. Suppressed emotions may rise to the surface in order to be eliminated. Your emotions could go up and down too, particularly if you are used to eating lots of refined foods full of sugar. These mood swings will soon pass. Try not to reach for comfort foods such as sweets and chocolate or cigarettes. Instead take flower remedies (see page 136) or use some aromatherapy oils (see pages 138 and 143).

Benefits of the detox

Rest assured you will soon feel absolutely wonderful as your body detoxifies.

Some of the many benefits include:

- Weight loss
- High energy levels
- Less or no cellulite
- Smooth, glowing skin
- Less stress and tension
- Clear headedness
- Positive state of mind
- Improved concentration
- Shiny lustrous hair and strong nails
- No bloating, flatulence, diarrhoea, constipation or indigestion
- Fewer or no aches and pains
- Healthy immune system with far fewer coughs and colds
- No headaches
- Deeper and more restful sleep
- No mood swings
- Fresh, sweet-smelling breath.

I hope that the promise of just a few of these many benefits will inspire you to detox!

Items you will need

Prior to commencing the programme it is important to gather all the items around you that you will need for your detox. If you have them ready to hand this will make your daily routine smoother and simpler.

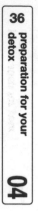
Not all of the items are compulsory and if you do not have every item then you will find you can improvise quite well if you use a little imagination.

Checklist

- Steamer
  This is to steam your vegetables as well as your fish. If you boil vegetables then most of the precious vitamins will be left in the water. You need these vital nutrients.

- Blender/Food processor
  A blender is ideal for making fresh fruit smoothies packed full of nutrients at breakfast time. It can also be used for blending delicious, healthy soups. A food processor will shred vegetables, in no time.

- Juicer
  Ready-made vegetable and fruit juices are available from supermarkets and health stores but they are often quite expensive. Also, some juices may have additives and preservatives in them and they may have been heated to high temperatures to pasteurize them to prolong their shelf life. Freezing is preferable to pasteurization, irradiation and canning, as although some vitamins and enzymes are lost during the process of freezing and thawing it is not as destructive as the other methods, which will be depleted of vitamins, minerals and enzymes. Enzymes are organic catalysts that increase the rate at which foods are broken down and absorbed by the body. They are found in plant foods such as fruits and vegetables and are unfortunately destroyed if you cook them. Invest in the best juicer that you can afford. You will quickly recoup the cost of a juicer and even after the detox you will find that you will want to make juicing part of your daily life. Juices are packed full of nutrients and will save you a fortune in vitamin and mineral supplements. Also you and your family will have lots of fun using the juicer.

  There are a wide variety of juicers available varying in price. The most inexpensive and popular juicers are centrifugal juicers and the more expensive are the masticating juicers which produce more juice. When shopping for a juicer consider practical factors other than the price. You do not want a machine that is too big and heavy and takes up most of your kitchen. How easy it is to clean? If it is time-consuming then you will not enjoy using it and it will soon be confined to the back of a cupboard.

If you are unable to buy a juicer then you can at least squeeze citrus fruits by hand.

- Thermoses
Thermoses are designed to retain both heat or cold. They are extremely handy for transporting cold nutritious juices to work in the summer as well as delicious warming soups and vegetable dishes. Since any contact with light, heat or air is detrimental to fresh juice and starts the process of oxidization, a thermos flask in the fridge is a superb way to extend the life of your fresh juice.

- Airtight food containers
It is advisable to have a variety of sizes. You can prepare fairly large quantities of food such as brown rice and soups and store them safely in your containers. They are also useful for transporting your lunches and snacks.

- Skin/Body brush
You will need a skin brush made from firm natural bristles. A brush that is too hard or stiff may irritate the skin whereas a soft brush will not effectively stimulate the circulation and lymphatic system. During your detox (and afterwards) it is an excellent idea to dry brush your skin every day (see page 94 for details).

- Tongue scraper
During a detox as your body eliminates the toxins you will find that a coating may accumulate on your tongue which can cause bad breath. To make your tongue look pink and healthy and to prevent halitosis, a tongue scraper is a good investment. You can purchase one from your dental practice or from your local pharmacist. It will really improve your oral hygiene. If you do not want to purchase a tongue scraper then you can use a soft toothbrush instead.

- Epsom salts
For best results during the detox you should take an Epsom salts bath every few days. This will help to speed up the elimination of toxins since Epsom salts are very effective at pulling toxins out of the skin. You can purchase them from larger chemist's and health-food shops. You will need two cups per bath.

- Bath/Shower
  During the detox you will be taking a bath/shower every day to speed up elimination.

- Somewhere to exercise
  Every day you will be taking 20 minutes of exercise. Do not worry – it is not necessary to join a gym. Clear a space in your bedroom or lounge, or the garden is the perfect place for exercise.

- Massage Oil/Cream
  During the detox it is advisable to carry out self-massage at least once a day to enhance the detox process. Preferably you need a cold-pressed vegetable, nut or seed oil. It should be unrefined, untreated by chemicals and additive free.

  Sweet almond oil is particularly popular but you can use virgin olive oil.

  Do not buy mineral oil which tends to clog up the skin whereas vegetable oils nourish the skin and contain vitamins, minerals and fatty acids. Massage techniques are explained on page 99. Aromatherapy oils are also described in this book as a way of accelerating your detox (see pages 122–6).

- Natural deodorant stone
  Whilst you are detoxing, your sweat glands will be working overtime and to begin with you may find that you are a little smellier (especially in the armpit area!) than usual. Do not block up the pores with an antiperspirant deodorant. You want those toxins out!

  Instead try to purchase a natural deodorant stone. They are 100 per cent pure and natural and are made from mineral salts extracted from natural mineral springs crystallized over a period of months. They are cut and shaped into approximately a 126 gram stone which looks rather like a clear bar of soap! Such a stone is highly economical and lasts from six months to a year. You are not putting any harmful chemicals or perfumes into your body and there is no aluminium chloride (found in many deodorants), which may be involved in Alzheimer's disease and certainly causes lymphatic congestion.

  Natural deodorant stones tackle the bacteria that are the cause of the odour. They prevent the bacteria from proliferating and no toxic residue is left behind – just a thin layer of mineral salts on the skin which cannot be felt or seen and which is not absorbed into the skin.

Natural deodorant stones are particularly recommended for individuals with sensitive skin since they are hypoallergenic and cause no irritation (see Useful addresses on page 175 for suppliers).

- Detox diary
  It can be most illuminating and also very amusing to keep a daily record of how you feel, not only physically but also emotionally, during your detox. Buy yourself an attractive notebook and write down any effects of the cleanse on your physical body and also any feelings that come up no matter how silly you may think these thoughts are. After all no one else is going to read it unless you publish your *Diary of a detoxer*! If you are experiencing negative emotions such as worry or thoughts about the past, this will allow you to release them. Negative emotions have a detrimental effect on our health. So let go of your emotional toxins as well as your physical congestion.

These are all the non-food items that you require. In the next chapter you will be making your food shopping list.

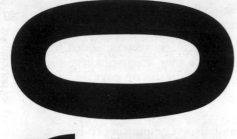
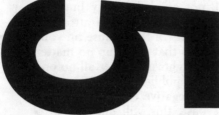

05 the food detox programme

In this chapter you will learn:
- about the advantages of eating organically
- about the foods and drinks permitted on the detox programme
- about foods and drinks to avoid whilst detoxing.

In this chapter we will be looking in detail at all the healthy, nutritious foods and drinks you will be enjoying during your 21-day detox. You will not be counting calories nor will you be starving yourself. In the 21-day plan you will be eating the most delicious, energizing foods you have ever tasted. This plan will make you look and feel so great that you will not want to go back to your poor dietary habits and unhealthy lifestyle.

After the detox if you adopt just a few of the dietary measures outlined in this chapter you will live a healthier life.

Try to eat organic

You can now find organic produce in the majority of supermarkets as well as in some health shops. By using organic food, you will be eliminating toxins from your diet since non-organic fruit and vegetables are routinely grown with the use of chemical fertilizers and pesticides – even our meat, fish and dairy foods are full of chemicals.

Unfortunately, organic foods are more costly but if you are able to stretch your budget then give them a try and notice how different they taste. Remember that organic food goes off more quickly than conventional fruit and vegetables due to the lack of artificial preservatives and so you will have to buy little and often.

However, if you do not wish to buy organic foods then this is perfectly acceptable. You will be eating lots of fresh fruit and vegetables throughout the detox, packed full of vitamins, minerals and fibre and these will give your system an enormous boost.

Cleaning your fruit and vegetables

Even if you decide to eat organic, you will probably find it difficult (and expensive) to obtain all the varieties of fruit and vegetables that you need. If you clean your produce carefully, you will be able to remove at least some of the pesticides and also most bacteria and parasites that are found even on organic foods.

You can simply rinse your produce thoroughly under the tap or if you wish to be extra careful try dipping them into boiling water for just a few seconds. Even more thorough is a lemon bath rinse:

- Fill a sink or a large bowl with cold water.
- Add a few tablespoons of salt together with the juice of a freshly-squeezed lemon.
- Place the fruit and vegetables into the lemon bath for five to ten minutes and then rinse thoroughly in cold water.

This is a marvellous way to destroy bacteria, parasites and agricultural chemicals.

Cooking your vegetables

Raw vegetables (as well as fruit) are incredibly nutritious and bursting with vitamins and minerals. Try to eat some raw food every day and when you cook foods try to remember the following:

- Cook vegetables as lightly as possible so that they have a firm texture. They should not be soft and soggy.
- Steaming is an excellent method of cooking.
- Stir frying is also a good alternative to boiling. Make sure that you only use a small amount of oil – preferably cold-pressed olive oil.

Fruit

Fruits form a valuable part of my detox plan. They are an invaluable source of antioxidants such as vitamin C, beta-carotene (the plant form of vitamin A), bioflavonoids as well as vitamin E. You may well have read in magazines and newspapers about nutraceuticals, phytochemicals and antioxidants but not understood what these words mean. Let me explain! Nutraceutical refers to foods or parts of foods that provide health benefits including preventing and treating diseases. For instance, fibre helps to prevent colon cancer. Phytochemicals and antioxidants are types of nutraceuticals. Phytochemicals (from the Greek *phyto* meaning 'plant') simply means 'plant chemicals'. Fruits (as well as vegetables) that are brightly coloured – for instance, red, orange and yellow – contain a great deal of phytochemical compounds. Some of the most important are the carotenoids and more than 600 carotenoids have been identified so far. They are responsible for the yellow, orange and red pigments that colour our fresh produce. Studies have revealed that these natural plant compounds can boost the immune system, decrease the risk of heart disease and hypertension and even protect against some cancers, as well as macular (retinal) degeneration.

Carotenoids include beta-carotene (converted to vitamin A in the body), which occurs for instance in yellow–orange foods such as apricots, mangos, melons, paw paws and carrots. Other carotenoids include alpha-carotene (also converted to vitamin A in the body), plentiful in carrots and pumpkins, thought to prevent lung cancer, and lycopene found especially in tomatoes which is thought to prevent prostate cancer.

Research shows that eating two or three servings of red, orange or yellow fruits a day, which are rich in carotenoids, can reduce the risk of cancer by 50 per cent.

Antioxidants include the carotenoids (such as betacarotene, the plant form of vitamin A, which is one of the best-known antioxidants), vitamin C, vitamin E, the minerals selenium, zinc and copper and also bioflavonoids. Antioxidants are said to 'mop up' free radicals. Free radicals are unstable oxygen molecules which are the natural by-products of many processes within, and among, cells.

Exposure to various environmental factors such as cigarette smoke and environmental pollution can also cause the body to produce free radicals. These free radicals can cause extensive cell damage and lead to diseases such as cancer, heart disease and even premature ageing. So, we really need our antioxidants to mop up the free radicals before they harm our bodies, and fruit (as well as vegetables) is an excellent source.

Fruit not only provides us with most of our vitamin C often along with bioflavonoids, beta-carotene, and in a small number of fruits vitamin E, but it is also a good source of potassium which helps to regulate blood pressure (especially dried fruits and bananas) and iron (found especially in dried fruit) which prevents anaemia. Fruit is also an excellent source of fibre. It contains both soluble and insoluble fibre. The skin of many fruits is an excellent source of pectin which is the soluble fibre that can help to lower blood cholesterol levels and reduce toxicity in the body by removing heavy metals. In order to get the most fibre from your fruit and vegetables do not peel them, although, as previously mentioned, it is essential to wash them thoroughly. It is the insoluble fibre that helps prevent constipation and during a detox we certainly need to do this! Fruit is also low in calories and therefore is ideal to promote weight loss.

You will notice in the breakfast recipes later in the book that fruit plays a major part. A light breakfast of fruit makes an ideal start to the day since it requires very little energy for digestion. A light breakfast will make you feel light, vibrant and energetic. A heavy breakfast will make you feel heavy and lethargic. Fruits are the cleansers and are perfect for a detox.

Shopping list

You may include as many fruits as you wish on your shopping list.

Eat a minimum of three portions of fruit per day (preferably raw). A portion is:

- One medium fruit (e.g. apple)
- Two small fruits (e.g. plums)
- One cupful of berries (e.g. raspberries)
- One large slice of large fruit (e.g. melon)
- One glass of pure fruit juice.

Main benefits of fruits

- Excellent source of antioxidants
- Reduce risk of cancer
- Prevent heart disease
- Boost immune system
- Prevent premature ageing
- Excellent source of fibre
- Excellent cleansers
- Source of potassium.

Apple
- Source of pectin (useful for absorbing toxins)
- Source of quercetin (an antioxidant)
- Source of potassium which helps to regulate blood pressure
- Source of vitamin C
- Excellent cleanser
- May help constipation as it improves bowel function
- Cleanses the liver

- Improves lung function
- Helps excrete heavy metals such as lead.

Apricot
- Source of fibre and beta-carotene
- Source of vitamin C
- Source of folic acid
- Dried apricots are a good source of iron, potassium and beta-carotene but avoid apricots treated with sulphur dioxide (preservative) which can trigger an asthma attack in susceptible individuals.

Avocado
- Source of glutathione which aids elimination of harmful fats
- Source of antioxidants (A, C, E), thought to prevent cancer, heart disease and anti-ageing
- Rich in monounsaturated fatty acids, thought to lower cholesterol
- Source of potassium, thought to regulate blood pressure
- Source of fibre
- Source of folic acid.

Banana
- Excellent source of potassium which helps to regulate blood pressure
- Source of phosphorus
- Source of magnesium
- Source of fibre.

Only eat ripe bananas since green bananas are difficult to digest and cause wind.

Bilberry
- Source of antioxidants
- Source of fibre
- Stabilizes blood sugar levels.

Blackberry
- Source of fibre
- Source of antioxidants.

If you are allergic to aspirin, take care with blackberries as they contain salicylates which could cause hyperactivity.

Blackcurrant
- Source of antioxidants, especially rich in vitamin C
- Remedy for sore throats
- Remedy for bacterial stomach upsets.

Blueberry
- Source of antioxidants
- Source of fibre
- Stabilizes blood sugar levels
- Remedy for digestive upsets
- Remedy for cystitis.

If you are allergic, take care as blueberries can cause an itchy rash and swelling of the lips and/or eyelids.

Cherry
- Source of potassium
- Source of antioxidants
- Eliminates toxins
- Relieves constipation
- Prevents gout.

Cranberry
- Source of antioxidants
- Remedy for the kidneys and bladder
- Combats problems such as cystitis.

Dates
- Source of vitamin C (fresh dates are richer than dried)
- Source of potassium, iron, magnesium (dried dates are richer) – regulates blood pressure, prevents anaemia
- Excellent source of fibre exerting a gentle, non-irritating laxative action.

If you are susceptible to migraine then take care as dates can trigger an attack in susceptible individuals.

Fig
- Excellent source of fibre with a mild laxative effect
- Source of potassium, iron, calcium and magnesium.

Gooseberry
- Source of vitamin C
- Source of fibre.

Grape
- Source of potassium
- Source of bioflavonoids (red and black grapes)
- Anti-cancer, anti-ageing
- Cleanses the liver, bowel, kidneys and lymph.

Grapefruit
- Source of vitamin C
- Contains pectin that may lower blood cholesterol levels
- Source of bioflavonoids that may protect against cancer
- Pink/red grapefruit (as opposed to white) provides an excellent source of vitamin A.

Guava
- Source of vitamin C
- Source of fibre
- Source of potassium
- Cleanses the liver and bowel.

Kiwi fruit
- Source of antioxidants (one kiwi supplies more than the adult daily requirements of vitamin C)
- Anti-cancer, immune boosting, anti-ageing
- Source of potassium
- Source of fibre.

Kumquat
- Source of antioxidants
- Source of fibre.

Lemon
- Source of vitamin C
- Detoxifies the liver
- Stimulates detox enzymes
- Cleanses the lymph
- Lowers cholesterol
- Counteracts acidity
- Immune boosting.

Lime
- Source of vitamin C
- Source of bioflavonoids to protect against cancer
- Immune boosting.

Lychee
- Source of vitamin C.

Mango
- Source of vitamin C
- Source of fibre
- Excellent source of beta-carotene
- Anti-cancer
- Source of potassium
- Cleanses the liver and bowel.

Melon
- Source of vitamin C
- Source of beta-carotene (cantaloupe melon is a superb source)
- Source of potassium
- Detoxifies the liver and bowel.

Nectarine
- Source of vitamin C
- Source of beta-carotene
- Source of potassium.

Olive
- Prevents heart disease
- Anti-cancer
- Source of beta-carotene
- Source of vitamin E.

Orange
- Source of vitamin C (one orange provides the adult daily requirement)
- Source of antioxidants
- Source of fibre
- Anti-cancer
- Immune boosting.

Papaya (paw paw)
- Source of vitamin C (half a fruit provides the adult daily requirement)
- Cleanses the liver and bowels
- Source of beta-carotene
- Source of potassium
- Source of fibre.

Passion fruit
- Source of antioxidants.

Peach
- Source of vitamin C (one peach supplies three quarters of the daily requirement of vitamin C)
- Source of fibre
- Gentle remedy for constipation
- Source of beta-carotene
- Anti-cancer.

Pear
- Source of vitamin C
- Source of pectin
- Source of antioxidants
- Source of potassium
- Source of fibre
- Cleanses the liver and bowel.

Persimmon (Sharon fruit)
- Source of vitamin C
- Source of beta-carotene
- Source of potassium.

Pineapple
- Source of vitamin C
- Aids digestion (contains bromelain)
- Combats sinus congestion and catarrh
- Source of potassium
- Cleanses the bowel and liver.

Plum
- Source of beta-carotene
- Source of vitamin C
- Source of fibre
- Source of potassium
- Cleanses the bowel and liver
- Anti-cancer.

Pomegranate
- Source of vitamin C
- Source of fibre if you eat the seeds
- Cleanses the bowel and liver.

Prune
- Source of fibre
- Remedy for constipation
- Source of potassium
- Source of iron – prevents anaemia.

If you suffer from flatulence when you first eat prunes don't worry, this will subside once your body gets used to them.

Raisin
- Source of potassium
- Source of fibre
- Source of iron.

Raspberry
- Source of vitamin C
- Source of antioxidants
- Boosts immune system
- Source of fibre
- Cleanses the liver, kidneys, lymph and bowel.

Redcurrant
- Source of antioxidants
- Source of potassium.

Strawberry
- Source of vitamin C
- Cleanses the digestive system
- Tonic for the liver.

May cause allergic reactions (hives). Avoid if you are allergic to aspirin. Avoid if you have a bowel disorder, since the seeds may be an irritation.

Tangerine
- Source of beta-carotene
- Source of vitamin C.

Tomato
- Source of beta-carotene
- Source of lycopene, thought to prevent prostate cancer
- Source of potassium
- Reduces the risk of heart disease
- Anti-cancer.

May cause mouth ulcers in susceptible individuals.

Watermelon

- Source of fibre
- Source of antioxidants
- Cleanses the liver and bowel.

Vegetables

Vegetables are an invaluable source of fibre, vitamins and minerals. Studies reveal that diets that are rich in vegetables (and fruit) prevent the risk of cancer. The cruciferous vegetables which include broccoli, Brussels sprouts, cauliflower, cabbage, bok choi and kale, are particularly linked with a lower risk for lung, stomach, colorectal, prostate and bladder cancer. Vegetables are also powerful antioxidants, neutralizing free radicals and preventing heart disease and premature ageing. Many vegetables are rich in carotenoids. The darker green the vegetable is, the higher the nutrient content. Vegetables are a good source of fibre, which helps to prevent constipation. You should eat a minimum of three portions daily – perhaps include a salad at lunchtime and some cooked vegetables for your evening meal.

Shopping list

You may include as many vegetables as you wish in your shopping list.

Eat a minimum of three portions per day. A portion is:

- Two tablespoons of raw/cooked vegetables, e.g. broccoli
- One dessert bowl of salad, e.g. lettuce.

Main benefits of vegetables

- Prevent the risk of cancer
- Source of antioxidants
- Source of fibre
- Source of folic acid
- Source of potassium
- Detoxifying.

Artichoke
- Source of fibre
- Source of folic acid
- Source of antioxidants
- Source of potassium
- Detoxifies the liver
- Lowers cholesterol
- Detoxifies the bowel
- Cleanses the blood and lymph.

Asparagus
- Source of folic acid
- Source of potassium
- Source of vitamin C, vitamin E and beta-carotene
- Cleanses the liver, bowels, kidneys and lymph.

Aubergine
- Source of fibre
- Source of folic acid
- Source of potassium
- Source of beta-carotene
- Lowers cholesterol
- Cleanses the liver and bowel.

Bean (Green)
- Source of beta-carotene
- Source of vitamin C
- Source of folic acid
- Source of fibre
- Cleanses the liver and bowel.

Beetroot
- Leafy tops are a source of beta-carotene, calcium and iron
- Source of folic acid
- Source of potassium
- Source of fibre
- Source of vitamin C
- Aids bowel function
- Cleanses the liver and blood.

Broccoli
- Excellent source of beta-carotene
- Source of vitamin C
- Source of folic acid, iron and potassium

- Source of fibre
- Source of indoles which can deactivate cancer cells
- Increases levels of detox enzymes
- Detoxifies liver and bowel.

Brussels sprout
- Source of fibre
- Source of indoles
- Assists the liver to get rid of toxins
- Detoxifies the bowel
- Source of vitamin C
- Source of iron
- Source of beta-carotene
- Source of folic acid
- Source of potassium.

Cabbage
- Source of fibre
- Source of potassium
- Source of folic acid
- Source of beta-carotene
- Source of vitamin C
- Detoxifies the liver, bowel and kidneys
- Protects against cancer.

NB Green cabbage contains most nutrients.

Carrot
- Excellent source of beta-carotene
- Source of fibre
- Source of potassium
- Eliminates putrefactive bacteria in the colon
- Source of iron and calcium
- Protects against cancer
- Cleanses the liver
- Good for healthy skin and eyesight.

Cauliflower
- Source of potassium
- Source of antioxidants
- Source of fibre
- Protects against cancer
- Cleanses the liver and bowel.

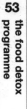

Celeriac (celery root)
- Source of potassium
- Source of fibre
- Source of antioxidants.

Celery
- Source of potassium
- Cleanses the kidneys
- Cleanses the liver, bowel and blood
- Relieves gout.

Courgette (zucchini)
- Source of folic acid
- Source of fibre
- Source of potassium
- Source of beta-carotene
- Source of antioxidants
- Cleanses the liver and bowel.

Cucumber
- Reduces water retention
- Source of beta-carotene (skin)
- Source of potassium
- Cleanses the liver, bowel and kidneys.

Fennel
- Source of folic acid
- Source of antioxidants
- Source of potassium
- Aids digestion
- Detoxifies the liver
- Cleanses the bowel, kidneys and blood.

Kale
- Source of vitamin C
- Excellent source of beta-carotene
- Source of fibre
- Protects against cancer
- Source of folic acid
- Source of iron, calcium and potassium
- Cleanses the liver and bowel.

Leek

- Source of fibre
- Source of potassium
- Source of antioxidants
- Aids the kidneys
- Cleanses the liver and bowel.

Lettuce

- Source of folic acid
- Source of beta-carotene (the darker the leaves the higher the source)
- Source of potassium
- Induces sleep
- Cleanses the liver, bowel and kidneys.

Mange tout

- Source of antioxidants
- Source of fibre
- Source of beta-carotene
- Source of potassium
- Cleanses the liver and bowel.

Okra

- Source of folic acid
- Source of potassium
- Source of beta-carotene
- Source of vitamin C
- Source of iron and calcium
- Cleanses the liver and bowel.

Onion

- Enhances healthy gut flora
- Reduces cholesterol
- Protects against cancer
- Prevents circulatory disease
- Source of potassium
- Cleanses the liver and bowel.

Parsnip

- Source of fibre
- Source of potassium
- Source of vitamin C
- Cleanses the liver and bowel.

Pea (fresh)
- Source of fibre
- Source of potassium
- Source of folic acid
- Source of phosphorus
- Source of beta-carotene
- Source of vitamin C
- Source of thiamine (vitamin B1)
- Cleanses the bowel and liver.

Pepper
- Source of vitamin C
- Source of beta-carotene (red peppers are the best source)
- Source of bioflavonoids
- Source of potassium
- Protects against cancer
- Reduces heart disease
- Cleanses the bowel and liver
- Boosts the immune system.

Potato
- Source of fibre
- Source of potassium
- Source of vitamin C
- Cleanses the bowel.

Pumpkin
- Source of beta-carotene
- Source of vitamin C
- Source of potassium
- Source of fibre
- Source of folic acid
- Protects against cancer
- Cleanses the liver and bowel.

Radish
- Source of vitamin C
- Protects against cancer
- Cleanses the liver, bowel and lymph.

Spinach (eat raw)
- Excellent source of beta-carotene
- Source of folic acid

- Source of vitamin C
- Source of iron
- Source of potassium
- Protects against cancer – especially colon
- Cleanses the bowel and liver.

Spring onion
- Source of fibre
- Source of vitamin C
- Source of potassium
- Cleanses the liver and bowel.

Squash
- Source of vitamin C
- Source of beta-carotene
- Source of fibre
- Source of potassium
- Source of folic acid
- Prevents cancer
- Cleanses the liver and bowel.

Swede
- Source of vitamin C
- Source of potassium
- Source of fibre
- Cleanses the liver and bowel
- Protects against cancer.

Sweetcorn
- Source of vitamin C
- Source of beta-carotene
- Source of potassium
- Source of phosphorus
- Cleanses the liver and bowel.

Sweet potato (yam)
- Excellent source of beta-carotene
- Source of fibre
- Source of potassium
- Balances blood sugar levels
- Source of vitamin C
- Cleanses the liver and bowel.

Turnip
- Source of fibre
- Source of vitamin C
- Source of potassium
- Source of folic acid (tops)
- Cleanses the liver and bowel.

Watercress
- Excellent source of beta-carotene
- Source of vitamin C
- Boosts the immune system
- Source of potassium
- Source of iron
- Cleanses the liver, bowel and lymph.

Sea vegetables (Seaweeds)

Sea vegetables, like land vegetables, are nutritious additives to our diet. Seaweeds are rich in minerals – for instance they contain 7–14 times more calcium than milk depending on the type of seaweed. They are also rich in iron, protein and fibre as well as vitamins A and C. They are most often associated with Japanese cuisine but they also frequently occur in Chinese and Korean cuisine.

Seaweeds are invaluable during a detox programme. They cleanse the intestines and also the lymphatic system and seaweeds are good for the immune system.

Below is a list of the varieties you may wish to try:

Arame
Arame is a good introduction to seaweed because of its mild taste. These dark brown, narrow, grass-like strands are often cooked with root vegetables such as yams and squash and served as a side dish.

Dulse
You may eat dulse raw as a snack or add it to salads. In Ireland it is added to mashed potatoes to create a dish called 'champ'.

Kombu
Kombu can be used to make soup stocks or can be cooked with rice or bean dishes. The recommended intake is 6.5 cm^2 size daily.

Nori

Nori (my favourite!) needs no cooking and is best known for being wrapped around sushi. You can wrap it around rice or simply sprinkle it into soups or over your food.

The recommended daily intake is one half to one sheet daily.

Wakame

Wakame are often cooked with soups. You can soak wakame, slightly blanch them or eat them raw. The recommended daily intake is a 6.5–13 cm^2 strip.

If you eat one portion of sea vegetables daily, this will boost your metabolism and enhance the detox. However, they are optional.

Grains

During the detox any products containing wheat are to be avoided. Sensitivity to wheat and its products is a fairly common phenomenon. In fact a large number of individuals with irritable bowel syndrome have an intolerance to wheat. Wheat is found in products such as bread and pasta, cereals, cakes, biscuits and pastry as well as in meat products such as sauces. It is also present in many processed foods as it is a cheap filler ingredient. Wheat allergy is not only responsible for the abdominal bloating, diarrhoea and/or constipation and flatulence found in irritable bowel syndrome but also it can be responsible for fatigue, headaches, weight gain, mental disturbances such as depression and anxiety, joint and muscular aches and pains, rheumatoid arthritis, headaches and skin problems such as eczema and psoriasis. It is thought that products that we eat too many of over a period of time, such as wheat, may cause our bodies to become allergic to them.

Some individuals are unfortunate enough to suffer from coeliac disease, which is intolerance to a protein called gluten. This is found not only in wheat but also in the grains oats, rye and barley. Most supermarkets nowadays stock a wide range of gluten-free foods as gluten intolerance is more widespread than you might think.

If you suffer with bowel problems then during the detox I would recommend excluding not only wheat but also oats, barley and rye. A good indication of food sensitivity is that you crave that food. Other common intolerances include certain nuts, especially peanuts, and also yeast, chocolate, cows' milk products, eggs, coffee, tea, soya, tomatoes, corn, shellfish, citrus fruits (especially oranges) and strawberries. You can be allergic to tap water and even to the plastic containers containing bottled spring water.

I recommend the following grains on the detox. They are rich in fibre, which helps to prevent constipation and is thought to reduce the risk of bowel disease. Whilst on the diet it is vital to keep the bowels working. Wholegrains also contain B vitamins, vitamin E and iron and they are excellent sources of carbohydrate and protein which help to boost our energy levels.

Shopping list

At least one portion daily.

Brown rice
Wholegrain rice is far superior to white rice that has been stripped of most of its fibre, vitamins and minerals. White rice also causes blood-sugar imbalances, mood swings and sugar cravings. If you think you may be intolerant then brown rice is an excellent choice for your detox. Brown rice has a wonderful cleansing effect on the bowels as it acts rather like a sponge absorbing and eliminating all the waste that is putrefying in your intestines.

Brown rice makes an excellent filling for vegetables such as red peppers and can be used as a base for a salad, wonderful curry or risotto. You can also enjoy rice cakes.

Buckwheat
Buckwheat flour can be used to make the Russian pancakes, blinis. Also try buckwheat flakes in cereals and buckwheat noodles in soups and in Japanese-style dishes.

Corn
Includes maize flour which can be used to make corn bread, popcorn, cornflour, corn pasta and corn chips and tortillas.

Millet (wholegrain or flakes)
Use wholegrain millet which can be boiled like white rice. Use millet flakes to make muesli, porridge or fruit crumble.

Quinoa
The grain is cooked like rice and the flakes can be used in breakfast cereals.

Barley, oats and rye

These grains contain gluten so avoid them if you think you may
be intolerant.

Pulses

Pulses (beans, peas and lentils) are highly nutritious and as they
are a good source of protein they are widely used by vegetarians
as an alternative to meat.

Pulses also contain both soluble and insoluble fibre. Soluble
fibre is thought to lower cholesterol whereas insoluble fibre
alleviates constipation and may provide protection against
bowel cancer. The starches in pulses are digested and absorbed
at a slow rate thus regulating blood-sugar levels as the glucose
is released steadily into the blood. Since they are digested slowly,
they make you feel full for longer. Pulses are a good source of
folate which may be useful in the prevention of diseases such as
heart disease and cancer. The phytoestrogens in pulses may play
a role in the prevention of hormone-related cancers such as
breast and prostate cancer. Pulses also provide B vitamins,
vitamin E, phytic acids and minerals such as iron, potassium,
magnesium, zinc and manganese. They have an added
advantage in being cheap and versatile and they are low in fat.

If you are cooking dried pulses, remember that you will need to
soak them overnight or for several hours prior to cooking.
Drain and rinse them and then cook them thoroughly. Be
particularly careful with kidney beans, which if raw or
undercooked can result in food poisoning.

You can use canned pulses but these have often been tinned in
salted water so you would need to drain and rinse them as salt
is not permitted on the detox plan.

Shopping list

If you are not used to eating pulses you are likely to become
flatulent so try not to overdo them to begin with! One portion
every two to three days is enough to get accustomed to them.

- Aduki beans
- Blackbeans
- Black-eyed peas
- Broad beans

- Butter beans (lima beans)
- Cannellini beans
- Chickpeas (main ingredient of hummus)
- Flageolet beans
- Kidney beans
- Lentils (red/green/brown) (no need to soak before cooking)
- Mung beans
- Pinto beans
- Soya beans
- Split peas (no need to soak before cooking).

Sprouts

Sprouts are one of the most complete and nutritional of all foods – they are nutritional superfoods. Their nutritional value was discovered thousands of years ago by the Chinese. Sprouts are fresh, living foods that amazingly continue to grow slowly and increase in vitamin content after you have harvested them. They are not like the fruit and vegetables that you buy in the supermarket that start losing their vitamin content immediately they are picked. They are superfoods rich in vitamins, minerals, proteins and enzymes and their nutrients are easy for the body to absorb.

Sprouted beans produce far less wind than whole beans and allergenic grains such as wheat and they do not induce an allergic reaction. Eating sprouted foods will help to keep your immune system strong, making you far less likely to become ill.

Sprouting is an excellent way to add more fresh and organic foods to the diet. There are no pesticides, preservatives or any of the other chemicals that are found on our produce nowadays. Growing your own sprouts is very cheap and it requires just a few minutes a day. Common seeds and beans for sprouting include alfalfa, peas, lentils, fenugreek, broccoli seeds, quinoa, millet, radish, pumpkin, mung beans, aduki beans and chickpeas. They make a nutritional addition to salads, sandwiches and soups. You can also fry them gently in olive oil and add them to casseroles and omelettes.

How to sprout your own!

You can buy a commercial bean sprouter or you can do it yourself with jam jars. Pick through a couple of handfuls of your chosen seeds or beans to discard any damaged ones. Place in a sieve and rinse thoroughly with plenty of water. Put them in a jar or bowl, cover them with water and allow them to soak for 12 hours or overnight in a warm, dark place.

Drain and rinse the seeds/beans and then place them in jam jars. Cover the jars with muslin or cotton secured with elastic bands and keep in a warm (approx 65°F, 17°C), dark place. If you wish, you can cover them with a dark cloth.

Rinse the seeds/beans twice every day, draining them thoroughly so that they do not become mouldy. You will have your fresh organic sprouts in just a few days' time.

Place the sprouts on a sunny windowsill for a few hours to give them a boost and they are ready to eat. You can store them in the fridge where they will keep for two to three days.

You can, if you wish, use a seed tray which you can line with moist kitchen roll. Place the soaked seeds on the lined tray and place in a warm, dark place. Then spray them twice a day with water.

Shopping list

If you decide to sprout your own then eat one portion daily. However, sprouts are optional.

- Alfalfa seeds
- Barley
- Blackbeans
- Broccoli seeds
- Buckwheat
- Brown rice
- Chickpeas
- Fenugreek
- Lentils
- Lima beans
- Millet
- Mung beans
- Mustard
- Oats
- Peas
- Pumpkin seeds
- Quinoa
- Radishes
- Sesame seeds

- Sunflower seeds
- Watercress
- Wheat.

Nuts and seeds

Most nuts and seeds have a high fat content which means that they are high in calories. For instance, ten walnuts contain about 250 calories and a tablespoon of sesame seeds 50 calories. An exception is the chestnut which is high in carbohydrate and low in protein and fat. However, do not think that nuts and seeds are bad for you! The fat in nuts is good for you as it is in the heart-healthy form of unsaturated fatty acids. Nuts and seeds help to lower blood cholesterol and prevent heart disease. The essential fatty acids, linoleic acid and alpha linoleic acid are particularly abundant in the majority of nuts and seeds. They are also rich in protein, fibre, the B vitamins, vitamin E, and the minerals iron, phosphorus, copper and potassium. Nuts should be eaten raw (vitamin E is destroyed when nuts are roasted) and unsalted. The best place to keep nuts is in the fridge or in an airtight container for they are prone to rancidity if they are exposed to light and air.

Shopping list

Try to eat a couple of tablespoons of nuts or seeds every day. Eat them on their own as snacks or add them to your smoothies, yoghurt and salads.

- Almonds (NB avoid eating immature almonds that can contain cyanide-producing compounds)
- Brazils
- Cashews
- Hazelnuts
- Linseeds (flaxseeds) – excellent for bowel health. Linseeds remove excess candida bacteria from the intestines. They also possess antibacterial, antifungal, antiviral and anti-cancer properties.
- Macadamias
- Pecans
- Pine nuts
- Pumpkin seeds – may help an enlarged prostate
- Sesame seeds (used to make halva and tahini which, when blended with chickpeas, makes hummus)

- Sunflower seeds
- Walnuts.

Fish

During the detox you will be avoiding all meat and meat products. Meat is difficult for humans to digest and meat putrefies in the intestines if the transition takes too long, producing poisons of a toxic nature to the body. This putrefaction of undigested food remnants leads to the formation of ammonia and other alkaline substances which paralyse the bowels. Apart from this, most meat contains antibiotics, hormones and other drugs. If you eat meat then organic free-range chicken would be the healthiest choice.

On the detox plan fish is allowed as it is a much more healthy choice. It is an excellent protein which is easily digested and is high in essential fatty acids and iodine which is required for the functioning of the thyroid gland. The omega-3 fatty acids found in fish help to protect against heart disease, reduce the risk of stroke and lower blood pressure. It is also thought that omega-3 fatty acids inhibit the progress of breast cancer and help to prevent tumours from occurring. Oily fish such as herring, mackerel, tuna, sardines and salmon are an excellent source of the omega-3 fatty acids and these fish are also rich in protein and vitamins A, B12 and D.

Whenever possible always choose fresh fish which contains the most nutrients. Wild fish, if available, is preferable provided the fishing area it comes from is not polluted. In fish farms chemicals are used to ward off parasites and colourings are sometimes added to feed to give the fish a pink colour. If no fresh fish is available then tinned fish preferably in olive oil or vegetable oil is acceptable. Do not choose fish in brine, which is salty and therefore not suitable for a detox plan. During a detox not only is fish high in nutrients but it also helps to reduce cravings.

Shopping list

Try to eat three to five portions of fish per week (oily fish is particularly beneficial) during the detox. Steam, bake or grill it with a nutritious salad or a plate of healthy vegetables.

- Bass
- Cod
- Haddock
- Halibut
- Herring
- Mackerel
- Monkfish
- Plaice
- Prawns
- Sardines
- Salmon (wild)
- Skate
- Sole
- Swordfish
- Trout
- Tuna.

Non-dairy foods

During the detox you should avoid all cows' milk products. If you crave milk and cheese it is likely that you have a sensitivity to dairy produce.

Milk increases the production of mucus in the body which is not beneficial during a cleanse. Interestingly many individuals who have an intolerance towards cows' milk products have no adverse reaction to goats' milk or sheep's milk products which are easier to digest. Cows' milk is not easily digested by humans. It generates unhealthy mucus which lodges in the sinuses and in the respiratory system in general. Indeed it is the most mucus-forming food that we can put in our bodies. If you suffer frequently from nasal problems, asthma or hayfever it is well worth giving up or drastically cutting down on dairy foods to see if your symptoms disappear. Some people have a lactose (milk sugar) intolerance and they experience symptoms such as abdominal bloating, wind, abdominal pains and diarrhoea.

Shopping list

Try to eat at least one portion daily.

- Almond milk
- Feta cheese

- Goats' milk
- Goats' milk yoghurt
- Goats' cheese
- Mozzarella cheese (made from buffalo milk)
- Oat milk
- Rice milk
- Soya cheese
- Soya milk
- Soya yoghurt.

Cold-pressed oils

Always use cold-pressed oils which provide essential fatty acids such as extra virgin olive oil, flaxseed and sesame seed. Omega-3 and omega-6 fatty acids are associated with a decreased risk of heart disease. Flaxseed oil is particularly rich in omega-3 essential fatty acids. Extra virgin olive oil is a marvellous antioxidant and is thought to be responsible for the health and longevity of those living in the Mediterranean area. Sesame oil is a good source of omega-6 fatty acids. Use these oils on their own or blend a couple together. If possible use unrefined organic oils.

Use your oils to make healthy salad dressings or pour over vegetables. You can also add them to juices and soups. Do not fry with these oils as high temperatures will reduce their nutritional value. Store your oils in the fridge to prevent them from going rancid. The following oils are highly recommended:

Shopping list

Try to have at least one tablespoon daily.

- Extra virgin olive oil
- Flaxseed (linseed)
- Pumpkin seed
- Rapeseed
- Sesame
- Sunflower
- Walnuts.

Culinary herbs and spices

Herbs and spices are highly recommended during the detox and indeed at all times. We really do not make use of them enough in our everyday diet. During the detox, replace salt with herbs and spices. Salt should be avoided as it is a preservative which makes food difficult to digest. It is also an addictive drug. High salt intake has been linked with high blood pressure, strokes and heart attacks. Excessive salt is stored in the body and results in waterlogged tissues such as cellulite and swollen ankles, wrists and hands. Salt is also indigestible, irritates the stomach and impairs the digestion of other foods. It is possible to get all the sodium salts we require from our fruit and vegetables such as asparagus, celery, spinach, kale, carrots, lettuce, spinach, strawberries and tomatoes. Instead of salt use herbs and spices to flavour your food. After salt has been omitted, you should really begin to enjoy the taste of your food more. Not only do herbs and spices enhance the flavour of your food but they have many health benefits too.

Here are a few herbs and spices that you may wish to introduce into your diet. If you are using fresh herbs then wash them carefully first to remove any pesticide residues:

Basil (sweet)
A wonderful tonic for the nervous system instilling peace and calm. It aids digestion and relieves stomach cramps. Basil is excellent if added to Italian dishes and essential for a tomato salad.

Bay
A tonic for the digestive system which expels wind and alleviates stomach cramps. Add bay leaves to your soups to give them flavour. (Bay is an ingredient of 'bouquet garni' together with parsley and thyme.)

Black pepper
A stimulating herb for the digestive system which helps to alleviate constipation. Black pepper effectively removes toxins from the system and provides pain relief.

Borage
A herbal remedy for the respiratory system, loosening phlegm and easing coughs. Use the leaves in your salads.

Caraway seeds

Caraway seeds help to relieve flatulence, abdominal bloating and colic.

Cardamom

A spice used in traditional Chinese and Indian medicine for over 3,000 years and recommended by Hippocrates. Use for stomach cramps, flatulence, constipation and indigestion.

Cayenne pepper

A wonderful herb with a multitude of uses. If you only try one herb get this! It is one of the most stimulating herbs known to humans which causes (surprisingly) no harm or reaction. In the West Indies it is widely used for all manner of illnesses and people chew and swallow the pods. It is excellent for constipation and as a general cleanser for the entire digestive system. Cayenne relieves flatulence, cramps and pains in the stomach and bowels. Sprinkle over your salads and soups.

Celery seeds

A good remedy for the liver which assists in detoxification and regeneration.

Chervil

Stimulates the whole digestive system. Chervil is cleansing and carminative, helping with flatulence and constipation. It is also a good remedy for the nerves, relieving depression and improving the memory. Add the leaves to salads and soups.

Chicory

Chicory can help to settle the stomach and is a cleansing herb and a tonic for the liver. Add it to your salads.

Chives

Tiny members of the onion family that help to stimulate the digestion. Add them to your soups, enliven your fish with them and sprinkle over your salads.

Coriander

A good stomach tonic that relieves flatulence and combats indigestion and spasm in the bowels. Use as a garnish, in soups, salads and curries. Good in ratatouille.

Dandelion

As a child, my mother told me not to sniff the dandelions otherwise I would want to go to the loo. There was an element of truth in it! Dandelion is a wonderful cleanser for the kidneys as well as the liver. Add a few leaves to a salad.

Dill

A cleansing herb that relieves flatulence and abdominal bloating. Delicious with fish dishes.

Fennel

Great for indigestion, flatulence, nausea and constipation and cleansing for the liver and gallbladder. If you chew fennel seeds not only will it settle your digestion but it also allays hunger. A good hormone balancer too. Add the feathery leaves to salads, vegetables and fish.

Fenugreek

Fenugreek enhances digestion and cleanses the digestive system. The leaves are a good addition to any salad.

Garlic

Garlic is a must-have that deserves a place in everyone's kitchen – not only during a detox. It is probably the most widely recognized of all herbs and is regarded as a miracle food. Garlic lowers blood cholesterol – one study showed that half to one clove of garlic daily lowered cholesterol on average by 9 per cent. It also reduces blood pressure and reduces the tendency of the blood to clot. Garlic is renowned for its ability to fight infection and boost the immune system. Garlic is antibacterial, antifungal and antiviral and kills off parasites in the intestines. It supports the beneficial flora of the intestines and combats yeasts and fungi such as candida.

Ideally you should eat one or two raw cloves of fresh garlic daily in your food to derive the maximum benefit. Cooking will decrease the nutritional value but is still acceptable. If you really cannot stand the smell then you can take odourless garlic capsules but you will lose some of its beneficial properties.

Ginger

Ginger is another of nature's miracles. It is one of the best spices for improving the digestion and has been used for thousands of years. Ginger is marvellous for relieving wind, pain and spasm in the digestive system. It is also a remedy for constipation and diarrhoea and well known for its ability to relieve nausea. It makes a wonderful tea. To make ginger tea, cut or grate a piece of fresh root ginger – enough to make two tablespoons of grated ginger. Place the grated ginger in a mug and pour over boiling

water. Leave to infuse for about ten minutes, strain it and it is
ready to drink.

Lemon balm

Lemon balm is one of the earliest known herbs and it is excellent
for calming the digestive system. Use for diarrhoea and
indigestion particularly if associated with the nerves.

Lemongrass

An excellent disinfectant for the digestive system which adds a
wonderful flavour to food. Use for Thai dishes and add to
soups, salads and curries.

Marjoram

A sedative herb that is an excellent tonic for the digestive
system. It has laxative properties and is a wonderful herb for the
alleviation of constipation. Marjoram also relieves flatulence
and indigestion. Add it together with basil and thyme to soups
and casseroles and use it in tomato sauces.

Mint

Widely recognized for its ability to aid digestion, mint is
soothing, eases pain and nausea and relieves gas in the stomach
and intestines. Great for bringing out the flavour of savoury
dishes and as an addition to salads.

Oregano

A traditional remedy for digestive upsets which has antitoxic,
antiviral and antibacterial properties. Oregano is a cleansing
herb that reduces wind and is a tonic for the digestive system.
Commonly called the 'pizza herb', oregano is great in Italian
dishes.

Parsley

An antioxidant, highly nutritious herb, containing iron and
vitamin C as well as potassium and vitamin A. Parsley helps to
detoxify the kidneys, liver and intestines. Use it with soups,
salads and fish. Fresh parsley can be chewed to freshen the
breath after eating garlic.

Rosemary

In use since ancient times for a wide variety of disorders,
rosemary cleanses the liver, gallbladder, kidneys and colon. It is
rich in antioxidants. Recommended for indigestion, flatulence,
constipation and to aid fat digestion. Use in salads, fish and
vegetables.

Sage

A herb with a history of use, sage was called the 'sacred herb' by the Romans. Sage is extremely cleansing and encourages the elimination of toxins. It can also relieve indigestion. Excellent in soups, risottos and in tomato sauces.

Thyme

A highly antiseptic herb, widely used since ancient times for medicinal purposes. It boosts the immune system and is a wonderful cleanser. Thyme gives soups and sauces an unmistakable flavour.

Turmeric

A well-known household spice used a great deal in curries. Turmeric is a source of antioxidants. It strengthens the digestion and decongests the liver and gallbladder. An excellent addition to soups and curries.

Drying your own herbs at home

It is great fun to grow your own herbs and you will gain the maximum benefit from freshly picked herbs. The fresher the herb the better! Any surplus may be dried so that you have your own organic herbs all year round!

As soon as you have picked your herbs make small bunches of them, hang them upside down, stems upwards, to dry. Place a large tray under the bunches or cover them with a paper bag to catch any falling dried material such as seeds. Once they have dried and become brittle, gently rub them off and store them in dark, airtight containers where you can keep them for up to 18 months. You can also chop herbs finely and place them in an ice-cube tray which you top up with water and freeze. About one tablespoon of herbs should fit into each ice cube – an ideal amount for a soup.

NB If you use dried herbs in cooking one teaspoon of dried herbs equals one tablespoon of fresh herbs.

Drinks

Coffee and tea

During the cleanse, coffee (including decaffeinated versions), tea and other drinks containing caffeine such as cola-based drinks should be avoided. Decaffeinated drinks are not acceptable because even though the caffeine has been removed they are often full of chemicals which are used in the process. Chocolate, unfortunately, also contains caffeine! An average cup of tea contains 50 mg of caffeine and a cup of coffee 100 mg, although it does vary depending on how strong your tea or coffee is. Adverse effects can be experienced from as little as 50 mg of caffeine and doses of 250 mg upwards (i.e. five cups of tea daily or just two to three cups of coffee) can produce significant effects such as:

- Excessive urination
- Diarrhoea, flatulence, indigestion and stomach upsets
- Headaches
- Palpitations and abnormal heart beat
- High blood pressure and elevated cholesterol
- Anxiety and nervousness
- Insomnia
- Depression
- Restless or jumpy legs, particularly troublesome at night
- A tendency towards benign breast cysts
- Drinking tea and coffee at meals impairs iron absorption by one third and also inhibits zinc absorption.

You may be surprised by some of the symptoms such as the restless legs at night. I find with my patients that this is a very commonly experienced syndrome that is easily rectified! Also, if women suffer with painful or lumpy breasts they are surprised at the improvement when they give up or drastically cut down on tea and coffee.

If you drink numerous cups of tea or coffee don't just suddenly stop! Cut down gradually, reducing your intake initially by half – you should try to do this prior to the cleanse. A sudden withdrawal from caffeine will cause the most unpleasant headaches and you may feel aggressive. If you withdraw slowly you should experience no more than a mild headache. If you can wean yourself off tea and coffee it is well worth the benefits. You will be much less nervous and irritable and more energized. Once you reduce your intake you'll be very aware of the adverse effects your tea and coffee drinking was having on you. I find I am unable to drink coffee at all (just a few sips give me palpitations!) and if I drink a cup of strong tea I experience an instant headache!

Avoid alcohol

Alcohol is also not permitted on a detox. Prior to your cleanse I urge you to reduce your alcohol consumption by half to prevent withdrawal symptoms such as irritability and insomnia. Alcohol has detrimental effects on our nutrients, particularly the B vitamins as well as folic acid, calcium, magnesium, zinc and the essential fatty acids. Alcohol also increases our urine output and some people are allergic to alcohol. Alcohol does not contribute any essential nutrients to the diet (only calories which are converted to fat!) and increases our requirements for many nutrients. This may not be a problem for the moderate drinker if they have a good diet and are getting the correct nutrients from other sources. However, those who drink more heavily tend to not eat regularly or properly so the toxic effects of the alcohol are compounded by lack of nutrition. Excessive alcohol consumption can lead to high blood pressure, brain damage, cirrhosis of the liver, and an increased risk of gout and even cancer of the liver, oesophagus, larynx and mouth. Women who drink during pregnancy are putting their children at risk of mental retardation. I suggest that after the detox you should take care to drink alcohol only in moderation. One or two glasses of a good organic red wine in the evening or, if you prefer, a pint of additive-free beer can help to relax you. Have one or two alcohol-free days per week.

Drink water

During the detox you will need to drink plenty of water. You should aim for 2 litres of water per day and if you really can't manage this, 1.5 litres. You will be drinking a glass of water with a squeeze of fresh lemon first thing in the morning to help to detox your liver and to give your body a kickstart. Drink your water at regular intervals throughout the day rather than gulping down large amounts in one go (which puts pressure on your internal organs) and always carry a bottle of water with you. A good indicator that you are drinking enough is the colour of your urine which should be a pale yellow colour – not cloudy or dark in colour. It will take a few days to accustom your body to the increase in water and it will seem as if you are always going to the toilet! However, your body will soon adjust and you will become aware of how much better you feel. Aim to drink one glassful every hour. Avoid drinking too much water late at night or you will disturb your sleep as you will have to go to the toilet. You should also not drink too much water at meal times as it dilutes the digestive enzymes.

You will be amazed at how much better drinking the right amount of water can make you feel and the benefits are evident in just a few days. The majority of us are actually chronically dehydrated (90 per cent of the population) and experience symptoms such as tiredness, headaches, dizziness, dry skin, urinary infections, stress, inability to concentrate, slow metabolism, weight gain, cellulite, toxicity, aches and pains and high blood pressure. If you have any of these symptoms then just drinking water could improve your health. Lack of water is the number one cause of tiredness and simply five glasses of water daily can decrease our risk of colon cancer, breast cancer and bladder cancer. A mere 2 per cent drop in hydration will affect your concentration.

During the detox drink filtered bottled water if possible (still is preferable to fizzy). In emergencies you can use tap water but it is better to filter it. Natural mineral water is full of nutrients including calcium, magnesium, sodium, potassium, chloride, bicarbonates and sulphates.

If the only thing you do after the detox is to carry on drinking your 2 litres of water your quality of life and health will be improved enormously.

Herb teas

Herbal teas are permitted on the detox and they make a good alternative to tea and coffee. They are well known for their medicinal uses and their benefits have been harnessed for thousands of years. Some herb teas supply nutrients, like parsley for example, which supplies iron, others relieve nausea and indigestion, like peppermint, whereas others such as camomile relieve insomnia. Here is a list of some of the more popular herbs found in commercial teabags. Purists say that these are not as good as making your own using home-grown or freshly-dried herbs. However, ready-made teabags are convenient and readily available from supermarkets and health stores. Amongst the best brands (although more expensive) are Dr Stuart's botanical teas.

Camomile tea
- Calms the nerves
- Dispels anger and irritability
- Relieves insomnia
- Soothes the stomach
- Aids digestion.

Camomile tea is an acquired taste – you either love it or hate it. You can add a spoonful of honey if you do not like the taste of camomile.

Cinnamon tea

- Improves circulation
- Great for colds
- Relieves stomach upsets
- Stimulates digestion.

Dandelion tea

- Improves liver function
- Excellent for the kidneys, gets rid of excess fluid.

Elderflower tea

- Cleanses the systems
- Boosts the immune system
- Eases catarrh, sinus problems and hayfever.

Fennel tea

- Relieves stomach cramps
- Eases wind and bloating
- Cleanses the liver and gallbladder
- Combats constipation.

Ginger tea

- Improves digestion
- Relieves nausea
- Improves circulation
- Expels gas
- Eases stomach cramps
- A great pick me up
- Warming for colds and flu.

For details on how to make a mug of ginger tea see page 70.

Lemon tea

- Combats acidity
- Boosts the immune system
- Refreshes and revitalizes
- Detoxifies the liver.

Lemon balm (melissa) tea
- Eases tension and relaxes the nerves
- Relieves digestive problems
- Lifts the spirits.

Nettle tea
- Cleanses the blood
- Improves liver function
- Stimulates kidney function
- Reduces allergic reactions.

Peppermint tea
- Relieves bloating
- Eases constipation
- Excellent for the liver and gallbladder
- Combats nausea
- Useful for headaches
- Reduces wind.

Raspberry leaf tea
- Soothes the digestive tract
- Combats diarrhoea
- Rich in vitamins and minerals
- Eases menstrual discomfort.

Rosehip tea
- Rich in vitamin C
- Boosts the immune system
- Prevents bladder infections.

Rosemary tea
- Cleanses the liver and gallbladder
- Relieves aches and pains
- Combats indigestion, wind and constipation
- Improves circulation.

Sage tea
- Calms the nerves
- Stimulates elimination of toxins
- Improves digestion
- Relieves lung congestion.

St John's Wort tea
- Relieves anxiety and irritability
- Combats depression
- Uplifts the spirits.

Strawberry leaf tea
- Soothes the digestive tract
- Relieves diarrhoea.

Thyme tea
- Boosts the immune system
- Cleanses the systems
- Eases coughs, sore throats and catarrh.

Valerian tea
- Relieves insomnia
- Calms the nerves
- Eases stomach cramps.

Detox teas

There are also a number of commercially prepared detox teas available that contain a blend of detoxifying herbs. Some of the most popular herbs used in these herbal formulations include:

Burdock root
- Skin and blood cleanser
- Enhances liver function
- Diuretic.

Cascara
- Mild laxative
- Good for the liver and gallbladder.

Cayenne
- Purifies the blood
- Encourages detoxification
- Increases fluid elimination and sweating.

Dandelion
- Cleanses the blood
- Detoxifies the liver and gallbladder
- Diuretic
- Prevents constipation.

Echinacea
- Boosts the immune system
- Cleanses the lymphatic system
- Helps to destroy fungal, viral and bacterial infections
- Feeds the beneficial bacteria in the intestines.

Garlic
- Blood cleanser
- Natural antibiotic
- Lowers cholesterol
- Reduces high blood pressure.

Ginger root
- Stimulates circulation
- Induces sweating.

Goldenseal root
- Cleanses the blood, liver, kidneys and the skin
- Regulates bowel function
- Boosts the immune system
- Encourages detoxification.

Licorice root
- Mild laxative
- Detoxifies and balances the liver
- Detoxifies the kidneys.

Milk thistle
- Best known tonic for the liver (in Germany milk thistle is prescribed by physicians for liver disorders). Silymarin, the active compound in milk thistle, is one of the most potent liver protectors known. It helps to repair and regenerate the liver.

Parsley leaf
- Cleanses the kidneys
- Combats fluid retention.

Making your own herbal teas

There is nothing quite like making your own herbal teas either from freshly-picked herbs or dried herbs. It is surprisingly easy to do.

You will need:

- Teapot (must be glass, porcelain or earthenware as some metals react with the herbs)
- Strainer (or you can use a tisane cup which has its own strainer and lid).

To make an infusion (infuse = to steep without boiling)

Method (leaves and flowers):

- Dried herbs – use one teaspoon per cup of water
- Fresh herbs – use three teaspoons per cup of water.

1 Warm your teapot to prevent the tea from cooling down too quickly.
2 Place your leaves, stems or flowers in your warm teapot (or warm tisane cup) and pour over water that is just off the boil.
3 Cover and leave to infuse for ten minutes to allow the herbs' therapeutic properties to be released.
4 Strain the tea into a cup.
5 Strain any remainder into a cup, cover and store in a refrigerator and use within 24 hours of brewing.

To make a decoction (extract flavour by boiling)

Method (roots/bark/seeds):

You will need:

- Saucepan
- Knife (for roots)
- Spoon or pestle and mortar (for seeds)
- Strainer.

1 Cut the roots or bark into small pieces or if you are using seeds then 'bruise' them with the back of the spoon or a pestle and mortar.
2 Place 15g–30g of your chosen herb into a saucepan with approximately 500 mls (two cups) of cold water. Bring to a gentle boil, reduce heat and simmer gently for approximately 10–15 minutes according to your taste.
3 Strain into a cup.

A combination

To prepare a tea using both roots/bark/seeds together with leaves/flowers, first of all make your decoction using just your roots, bark or seeds. Then strain it and pour the strained decoction over your leaves or flowers and infuse as above.

Herbal iced teas

Follow the same directions as indicated above but make a double-strength brew. Strain and chill for approximately 30 minutes. Then pour over a glass full of ice.

Home-made teabags

Place one to two teaspoons of herbs onto a muslin square. Pull the corners together to make a small bag and tie up with string.

Have fun with these recipes!

Other permitted teas

Rooibos tea

Rooibos, also known as Rooibosch (old Dutch spelling), or 'Red bush', comes from the young shoots of a South African shrub. The plant is green until it is fermented, when it becomes red. It contains no caffeine, colours, additives or preservatives and it does not have a negative effect on the absorption of iron (as regular tea does). According to studies carried out in South Africa and Japan, it can help to relieve digestive problems such as stomach cramps (it is thought to be antispasmodic), allergies such as hayfever, eczema, asthma and irritated skin and nervous problems such as irritability and tension. It is also thought to slow down the ageing process. Rooibos tea is packed with nutrients including iron, calcium, magnesium, manganese, zinc and potassium. It contains no oxalic acid, making it a healthy beverage for people suffering from kidney stones.

You can pour boiling water over Rooibos tea and drink it hot. Another popular way of enjoying it is to make the tea, allow it to cool and pour it into a glass filled with ice, squeeze in the juice of half an orange and enjoy it cold.

Green tea

Green tea has been used as a medicine in China for at least 4,000 years. It is thought that a compound in green tea, known as EGCG (epigallocatechin gallate), reduces the growth of cancer cells. A Japanese report stated that men who drank ten cups of green tea per day stayed cancer free for three years longer than those drinking less than three cups. Japanese scientists have also revealed that there were less recurrences of breast cancer and it spread more slowly in women who drank five cups or more of green tea daily. Green tea is also reputed to lower cholesterol levels and reduce the incidence of heart disease due to the presence of the EGCG compound.

Green tea is also thought to help dieters and even prevents tooth decay as it has the ability to kill the bacteria causing tooth decay. Even skin preparations containing green tea are beginning to appear. Green tea, unfortunately, does contain caffeine albeit much less than regular tea or coffee (30 mg in green tea as opposed to 100 mg in a cup of coffee). The advantages of green tea outweigh this one drawback and provided you do not overdo the green tea in the evenings I am sure you will not suffer from insomnia.

Do not over brew your green tea or you will ruin the flavour. Allow it to steep for just three minutes and if you have used a teabag remove the bag. If you are using loose tea then you will need one to two teaspoons per cup of tea.

Dandelion coffee

For a coffee substitute, as a treat you could try dandelion coffee. It is made of high-quality roots which are dried and roasted. It has no caffeine so it can be drunk before bedtime. Although roasted dandelion contains many nutrients it should be remembered that any burned or browned food is to some extent carcinogenic. Therefore, even dandelion coffee should only be drunk in moderation.

Pure fruit and vegetable juices

The ability of fresh fruit and vegetable juices to cleanse and rejuvenate has been recognized for a long time. Juice making used to be a very tedious process involving the squeezing of crushed or chopped fruit and vegetables through muslin. Thankfully, due to the arrival of affordable centrifugal juicers which are so much easier to clean than the first juicers, it is easy to bring the benefits of fresh fruit and vegetable juices into our homes (the benefits of fresh juices versus store-bought juices are discussed on page 36).

Famous doctors such as Max Gerson (famous for his work with cancer) and Dr Bircher Benner have advocated juice therapy for their sick patients; some of whom had been given no hope to live. Fresh fruit and vegetable juices have actually saved some people's lives when they have undertaken juice therapy.

The juice of fresh fruit and vegetables provides a rich source of vitamins, minerals and enzymes (see pages 44–58 for details of the nutritional content of fruit and vegetables). In fact, nothing is more nutritious than juice! You can think of juices as powerful nutritional supplements.

If you drink juices on a regular basis you will never need nutritional supplements or vitamin and mineral supplements. It is difficult to eat the right amount of raw fruit and vegetables to nourish our bodies sufficiently, particularly when there are so many toxins from the environment, etc. and most of us do not have enough time. It would be difficult for you to eat half a kilo of carrots in one go but easy to drink a single glass of carrot juice! I am not trying to suggest that one should only drink juice and not bother with the raw, fruit/vegetables because you would miss out on nutrient such as fibre. We need fresh fruits and vegetables *and* fresh juices. For optimum health, eat three portions of fruit, three portions of vegetables and drink two glasses of juice (one fruit and one vegetable) every day. You will feel rejuvenated, your minor ailments will disappear and you will look much younger than your years (without cosmetic surgery!).

Some juicing tips

- Use organically grown, unsprayed produce.
- Always wash your produce well (see pages 41–2).
- Always peel oranges and grapefruits prior to juicing as they contain a toxic substance.
- If the produce has been waxed (e.g. lemons and limes) remove the peel. Otherwise you can leave on the peel of unwaxed lemons.
- Peel tropical fruits such as kiwi and papaya which have often been sprayed.
- Remove stones (e.g. plum stones) before juicing.
- You may put seeds in the juicer (but not apple seeds which contain small amounts of cyanide).
- You may juice stems and leaves – but not carrot or rhubarb leaves.
- Some fruits and vegetables are non-juiceable. It is only possible to juice produce which has a high water content. The non-juiceables include banana, coconut, avocado, prunes and other dried fruits. You may be thinking to yourself 'but I have enjoyed banana and apple juice at my local juice bar'. What has happened is that the apple has been juiced first and then the juice has been transferred to a blender and this has been used to mix in the banana.

Some of my fruit juice favourites are:

- Apple and pear
- Apple, orange and ginger
- Apple and grape

- Apple, cranberry and grape
- Orange and grapefruit
- Watermelon
- Raspberries, blackberry and apple
- Apple, pear and pineapple.

Vegetable or vegetable/fruit combos include:

- Carrot and apple
- Carrot, celery and ginger
- Carrot and spinach
- Carrot, orange and green pepper
- Carrot, beets and green pepper
- Carrot, apple and alfalfa sprouts
- Carrot and cabbage
- Tomato, celery and pineapple.

Green juices include:

- Celery and spinach
- Celery, spinach, cabbage and ginger
- Spinach, cabbage, ginger and cayenne.

Try to drink one glass of fruit juice and one vegetable or vegetable/fruit combination or green juice daily. See Chapter 8 for details of juice as well as smoothie recipes.

The acid–alkaline balance

It is important to maintain the correct acid–alkaline balance in our bodies to ensure optimum health. Acids can cause problems such as the overproduction of mucus, tension in the nervous system, arthritis, rheumatism, digestive disorders and respiratory ailments.

Some foods are acid-forming whereas others are alkaline-forming. Our bodies are designed to eat a diet that is rich in alkaline-forming foods. By this I mean the end result in the body, once the food has been digested. This can be confusing as some foods that are acid (e.g. lemon) have an alkaline effect on the body once they are digested. Alkaline foods include the majority of fruits and vegetables whereas acid-forming foods include protein foods such as meat, poultry, game, fish, egg, shellfish and cheese as well as bread and all foods made from flour, all grains (except millet), most nuts and seeds and all forms of sugar.

I am not suggesting that your diet should be totally alkaline forming. For the majority of people, the ideal acid–alkaline balance of their food intake is 70 per cent alkaline and 30 per cent acid-forming foods. Most people's diets are more like 70–80 or even 90 per cent acid!

One way of maintaining the body's original acid–alkaline balance is to take organic apple-cider vinegar and/or lemon juice daily.

Select your first drink of the day

Organic apple cider vinegar/organic lemon juice

Hippocrates, the father of medicine, extolled the virtues of apple cider vinegar. It acts as a powerful intestinal cleanser, helps to combat arthritis and aches and pains and helps to maintain the body's crucial acid–alkaline balance.

1 Organic apple cider vinegar
   The best way to take organic apple cider vinegar is to place one tablespoon in a glass of warm water. You may add a teaspoon of honey if you find the taste too bitter. Drink this first thing in the morning. NB Do not use malts or any other type of vinegar which is damaging to the body.

2 Lemon juice
   Alternatively, to balance the body's pH, squeeze the juice of a fresh lemon into a cup of warm water. As well as balancing the pH, the lemon juice will also help to flush out your liver.

3 Organic cider vinegar and lemon
   If you wish you can combine the apple cider vinegar and lemon juice. Squeeze the juice of a lemon into a cup of warm water and add one tablespoon of organic apple cider vinegar and a teaspoon of honey if desired.

Summary of foods and drinks on the detox programme

Fruit

- Apples
- Apricots
- Avocados
- Bananas
- Bilberries
- Blackberries
- Blackcurrants
- Blueberries
- Cherries
- Cranberries
- Dates
- Figs

- Gooseberries
- Grapefruits
- Grapes
- Guavas
- Kiwi fruit
- Kumquats
- Lemons
- Limes
- Lychees
- Mangoes
- Melons
- Nectarines
- Olives
- Oranges
- Papayas
- Passion fruit
- Peaches
- Pears
- Persimmons
  (Sharon fruit)
- Pineapples
- Plums
- Pomegranates
- Prunes
- Raisins
- Raspberries
- Redcurrants
- Strawberries
- Tangerines
- Tomatoes
- Watermelons.

Eat three + portions a day. One portion is the equivalent of:

- One medium fruit (e.g. apple)
- Two small fruits (e.g. plums)
- One cupful of berries (e.g. strawberries)
- One large slice of large fruit (e.g. melon)
- One glass of pure fruit juice.

Vegetables

- Artichokes
- Asparagus
- Aubergines
- Beans (green)
- Beetroots
- Broccoli
- Brussels sprouts
- Cabbages
- Carrots
- Cauliflowers
- Celeriac
- Celery
- Courgettes
  (zucchini)
- Cucumbers
- Fennel
- Kale
- Leeks
- Lettuces
- Mange tout
- Okra
- Onions
- Parsnips
- Peas
- Peppers
- Potatoes
- Pumpkins
- Radishes
- Spinach
- Spring onions
- Squashes
  (winter)
- Swedes
- Sweet potatoes/
  Yams
- Sweetcorn
- Turnips
- Watercress.

Eat three + portions a day. One portion is the equivalent of:

- One dessert bowl of salad
- Two tablespoons of raw/cooked vegetables.

Sea vegetables (optional)

- Kombu – 6.5 cm^2 piece = one portion
- Nori – half to one sheet = one portion
- Wakame – one 6.5–13 cm^2 strip = one portion
- Arame – two tablespoons = one portion
- Dulse – two tablespoons = one portion.

One portion of sea vegetables daily will help to keep your metabolic rates steady and cleanse the intestines and lymphatic system.

Grains

- Brown rice
- Buckwheat
- Corn
- Millet
- Quinoa.

Also barley, oats and rye. As these contain gluten avoid if you think you may have an intolerance.

Eat at least one portion daily.

Pulses

- Aduki beans
- Blackbeans
- Black-eyed peas
- Broad beans
- Butter beans (lima beans)
- Cannellini beans
- Chickpeas (main ingredients of hummus)
- Flageolet beans
- Kidney beans
- Lentils (no need to soak)
- Mung beans
- Pinto beans
- Soya beans
- Split peas (no need to soak).

Eat one portion every two or three days until you become accustomed to them.

Sprouts

These are optional but remember that they are nutritional superfoods.

- Alfalfa seeds
- Barley
- Blackbeans
- Broccoli seeds
- Buckwheat
- Brown rice
- Chickpeas
- Fenugreek
- Lentils
- Lima beans
- Millet
- Mung beans
- Mustard
- Oats
- Peas
- Pumpkin seeds
- Quinoa
- Radishes
- Sesame seeds
- Sunflower seeds
- Watercress
- Wheat.

Eat one portion daily (optional).

Nuts and seeds

- Almonds
- Brazils
- Cashews
- Hazelnuts
- Linseeds (flaxseeds)
- Macadamias
- Pecans
- Pine nuts
- Pumpkin seeds
- Sesame seeds
- Sunflower seeds
- Walnuts.

Eat a couple of tablespoons daily as snacks or add to salads, soups, smoothies and yoghurt.

Fish

- Bass
- Cod
- Haddock
- Halibut
- Herrings
- Mackerel
- Monkfish
- Plaice
- Prawns
- Sardines
- Salmon (wild)
- Skate
- Sole
- Swordfish
- Trout
- Tuna.

Eat three to five portions of fish (particularly oily) per week.

Non-dairy foods

- Almond milk
- Feta cheese
- Goats' milk
- Goats' milk yoghurt
- Goats' cheese
- Mozzarella cheese (made from buffalo milk)
- Oat milk
- Rice milk
- Soya cheese
- Soya milk
- Soya yoghurt.

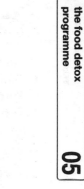

Eat at least one portion.

Cold-pressed oils

- Extra virgin olive oil
- Flaxseed (linseed)
- Pumpkin seed
- Rapeseed
- Sesame
- Sunflower
- Walnut.

Eat at least one tablespoon daily.

Herbs and spices

Use the folloing instead of salt.

- Basil
- Bay
- Black pepper
- Borage
- Caraway seeds
- Cardamom
- Cayenne pepper *
- Celery seeds
- Chervil
- Chicory
- Chives
- Coriander
- Dandelion
- Dill
- Fennel
- Fenugreek
- Garlic*
- Ginger*
- Lemon balm
- Lemongrass
- Marjoram
- Mint
- Oregano
- Parsley
- Rosemary
- Sage
- Thyme
- Turmeric.

* must haves

Drinks

- Water (aim for 2 litres daily)
- Herb teas
- Rooibos tea
- Green tea
- Dandelion coffee
- Pure fruit juice
- Pure vegetable juice.

If you have a juicer try to drink one glass of fruit juice and one vegetable or vegetable/fruit combination or green juice daily.

Foods and drinks to avoid

The reasons for avoidance of the following have been given throughout the book.

- Ready meals/ready-made sauces and salad dressings
- Processed and refined foods
- Salt (and any foods containing salt e.g. crisps)
- Sugar (and any foods containing sugar, e.g. chocolate, jam, biscuits, sweets, cakes)
- Artificial sweeteners (e.g. aspartamine)
- Wheat (and any foods containing wheat e.g. bread, cakes, biscuits)
- Meat
- Dairy foods.

Halve your intake of these drinks a few weeks prior to the detox to avoid unpleasant withdrawal symptoms.

- Coffee, tea and other caffeinated drinks
- Alcohol.

Your day-to-day detox summary

- On rising, drink one of the following:
  - a glass of warm water with lemon squeezed in

or

  - a glass of warm water with one tablespoon of organic apple cider vinegar (add one teaspoon of honey if desired)

- a glass of warm water with one tablespoon organic apple cider vinegar plus juice of squeezed lemon (add one teaspoon of honey if desired).
- Drink 2 litres of water during the day.
- Eat three meals daily, choosing permitted foods from the lists.
- Snacks should be healthy – fruit, raw vegetables, nuts, seeds, pure fruit or vegetable juices, smoothies.
- Eat three + portions of fruit daily.
- Eat three + portions of vegetables daily.
- Eat at least one portion of grains (e.g. brown rice) daily.
- Eat at least one portion of non-dairy foods daily.
- Eat at least one tablespoon of cold-pressed oils daily.
- Eat a couple of tablespoons of nuts and/or seeds daily.
- Eat one portion of pulses every two to three days.
- Eat three to five portions of fish (especially oily) per week.
- Use herbs instead of salt, especially cayenne, garlic and ginger.
- Eat one portion of sea vegetables (e.g. nori) to boost metabolism and detox (optional).
- Eat one portion of sprouted beans/seeds daily (optional).
- Drink one glass of pure fruit juice and one vegetable or vegetable/fruit combo daily (optional).

21-day food checklist

Why not complete the following checklist every day to see if you're keeping to the detox guidelines? You may wish to photocopy it and put it on your kitchen notice board.

Tick the boxes or fill in the number of portions you have eaten each day. If you only manage two portions of vegetables one day then aim for four the next day. If you eat five portions one day give yourself a pat on the back!

Day	1	2	3	4	5	6	7	8	9	10	11	12	13	14	15	16	17	18	19	20	21
Water + lemon/apple cider vinegar																					
2 litres water																					
3 x fruit (minimum)																					
3 x vegetables (minimum)																					
Grains (at least 1)																					
Non-dairy (at least 1)																					
Cold-pressed oils (at least 1 tbsp)																					
Nuts/seeds (at least 2 tbsp)																					
Pulses (every 2–3 days then increase)																					
Fish (3–5 portions weekly)																					
Herbs (not salt)																					
Sea vegetables (OPTIONAL)																					
Sprouted beans/seeds (OPTIONAL)																					
Juices (OPTIONAL)																					
Herb teas/Rooibos etc. (OPTIONAL)																					

06

the body detox programme

In this chapter you will learn:
- about the various techniques for detoxing the body.

This 21-day detox is not only about the foods you put into your body but also about ways of caring for your body that will assist the detoxification process. This is why on our checklist of items you will need there was a body brush, tongue scraper, Epsom salts, massage oils/creams and somewhere to exercise. My detox programme is holistic and this body detox programme should be carried out in conjunction with the food detox programme. The body detox treatments will greatly accelerate and enhance the process of detoxification. If you are going to detox then go for maximum effect!

Dry skin brushing

Dry skin brushing should be carried out every morning. It will take just a few minutes.

As we have seen, our skin is an organ of elimination just like our liver, kidneys, colon, lungs and lymphatic system. Good health is dependent upon our skin breathing and eliminating. We eliminate toxins via the skin through our sweat and more than 0.5 litres of waste products are discharged every day. The chemical analysis of sweat shows that it has almost the same constituents as urine! If our skin is inactive and its pores are clogged up with dead cells then the waste products such as uric acid will stay in our bodies. Then the liver, kidneys, lungs, colon and lymphatic system will have to compensate and work harder than ever. Eventually, they will become overburdened with toxins and disease will be the inevitable outcome. Thus, it is vital to skin brush. The many benefits include:

- More efficient and faster elimination of toxins
- The lymphatic system is stimulated so circulation improves
- Dead skin cells are removed, revealing healthy skin cells which make the skin glow
- The production of sebum, our natural moisturizer, is increased, resulting in soft, moisturized skin
- Fluid retention reduces
- Cellulite will diminish.

It is important to remember that skin brushing is performed on dry skin. So do not attempt it whilst you are in the bath or shower – always do it before. Dry skin brushing only takes about three or four minutes, so there are no excuses for not doing it every morning!

For best results, you will need a long handled skin brush made from natural bristles that are fairly firm but not so hard that they irritate the skin. A soft brush will not be effective as the brushing would not be firm enough to stimulate the systems of elimination. If you do not have a natural bristle brush then you can use a loofah, mitt or even a dry flannel, although a brush is best. Follow these instructions for best results:

1 Do not wet your body brush and do not use any moisturizer on your skin.
2 Take your clothes off and stand in a comfortable position where you will be able to reach all parts of your body easily.
3 Begin at the soles of your feet and brush the underneath and sides of your feet and/your legs making sure that you are completely covering the back, front and sides of them. Your strokes should be quite gentle to begin with but you can gradually increase the pressure after a few days for maximum benefit.
4 Now brush up the front of the body towards the heart, aiming for the armpits to assist lymphatic drainage. To stimulate your colon gently circle your brush over your abdomen in a clockwise direction so that you are following the colon.

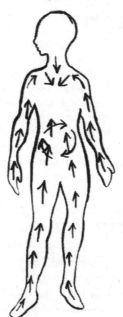

figure 2 direction of body brushing

5 Then brush the buttocks, up the back and towards the neck. Notice that we are always brushing towards the heart.

6 To brush your hands and arms, raise each arm (by elevating the arm, you are encouraging lymph drainage) and brush from the hand down, towards each armpit.

7 Finally, gently brush down the neck and down the top of the chest into each armpit.

NB Do not use your skin brush on your face as facial skin is extremely delicate. A soft dry flannel or a special soft facial brush could be used to remove the dead skin cells.

At the end of your skin brushing, your skin will tingle and feel warm as you have increased your circulation. Do not be alarmed if your skin looks red, as this is just the blood coming to the surface. Skin brushing makes the skin stronger so you can start to gradually apply firmer pressure. After skin brushing it is not uncommon to see mucus in the stools, which is a positive sign showing that the body is ridding itself of old toxins. Within days your skin will feel smooth and soft and will look healthy, toned and blemish free.

Hot/Cold showers

Follow your dry skin brushing routine with a hot shower and just before you have finished, switch the shower to cold for about 30 seconds. If you like a bath or do not have a shower take a hot bath as usual and empty out the water. Then run the cold tap and splash your body with cold water. You may not relish the idea of cold showers but they are extremely therapeutic. Regular cold showers improve the blood and lymph circulation. This improved circulation stimulates the elimination of toxins that have accumulated in the layers of fatty deposits. You will feel so much better after the toxins have been extracted from your body.

Cold showers also help to prevent and break down cellulite and they also decrease the likelihood of the formation of spider and varicose veins. As well as aiding detoxification cold showers also help you to lose weight. So be really brave in the mornings and turn the shower from hot to cold!

You may be thinking that cold showers are completely out of the question as they will make you feel too cold. On the contrary, a cold shower brings an immediate rush of blood through your system together with a rush of energy. This increased circulation makes you feel warm, invigorated, detoxified and toned!

Hot and cold water therapy is one of the techniques used in hydrotherapy. Hydrotherapy is the use of water in the treatment of disease and it is primarily employed to stimulate the circulation, the lymphatic and immune systems, the digestion and to provide pain relief. It also releases stress. Water therapy is an ancient therapy that has been practised for centuries by the ancients including the Greeks, Romans and Chinese. The healing properties of hydrotherapy exploit the reaction of the body to hot and cold stimuli. Hot water relaxes and soothes whereas cold water stimulates. Together, they are like a hydrostatic pump that makes the blood flow, resulting in better circulation. The cold water stimulates blood flow to the core of the body, bringing fresh blood to the internal organs, glands and all parts of the body and the hot water stimulates blood flow to the surface of the body. Thus oxygen and nutrients are drawn in and the toxins are pushed out.

Once you are feeling brave, try the following for an even more detoxifying and healthful effect:

1 Stand under the shower and slowly increase the temperature of the water so that it is as hot as you can tolerate it.
2 Turn the temperature down to the coldest bearable setting.
3 Now turn the temperature back to hot and see if you can make it even hotter than before. Then turn the shower down to cold again.
4 Repeat this hot–cold procedure seven times. Always end with cold water.

Try this procedure to really enhance the effectiveness of the detox programme. It will make you feel wonderful!

Tongue scraping

I have already said that one of the side effects of the detox in the early days is a coated tongue which can cause halitosis (bad breath). To counteract this, you may want to purchase a tongue scraper to ensure a lovely pink healthy tongue! You can easily obtain one from your dental practice or chemist's. Alternatively, use a soft toothbrush to gently clean away the toxic material. For extra cleaning, dip your toothbrush into warm water into which you have squeezed fresh lemon juice or even a cup of water with a few drops of essential oil of lemon and gently brush your tongue. Your breath will still feel fresh when you wake up in the morning.

Epsom salts baths

Epsom salts are made of magnesium sulphate, which is a natural occurring mineral. Epsom salts baths are excellent when on a detox as they draw toxins such as acidic wastes – mainly uric acid – out from the body through the skin. An Epsom salts bath is also a sedative for the nervous system and therefore helps to reduce stress. Other benefits include easing muscular aches and pains and relieving rheumatism and arthritis. It is also thought that an Epsom salts bath can counter the effects of low-level radiation thus combating VDU stress.

How to prepare an Epsom salts bath

You will need two cups of Epsom salts (this is approximately 450 g). You will not need to use any soap.

Simply run a full bath and add the salts to it, thoroughly agitating the water to fully disperse them. Relax in your bath for about 15 minutes. When you get out of the bath, wrap yourself up warmly to avoid becoming chilled. Try to rest for a couple of hours or even retire to bed early and enjoy a deeply relaxing sleep. During the detox it is a good idea to take an Epsom salts bath every three to four days to encourage detoxification.

Other Epsom salts uses

- You can also use your Epsom salts in a foot soak to relieve aches and pains, unpleasant odours and to soften rough skin. You will need half a cup of Epsom salts to a large bowl of water.
- Epsom salts can also be used as a skin exfoliator. Start at the feet (as with the dry skin brushing) and simply massage handfuls of Epsom salts into your wet skin. Then have a bath or shower to rinse.
- To cleanse your face mix half a teaspoon of water and Epsom salts with a natural cleansing lotion/cream. Massage your face gently and rinse off with cold water.

- To remove a splinter soak the affected area in a bowl of water with added Epsom salts and this will draw the splinter out.

Self-massage

A daily self-massage will greatly assist the detoxification process. You will be amazed at the benefits it offers for all the systems of the body:

- It accelerates the lymph flow helping to remove waste products from the system.
- It boosts the immune system, making us less prone to coughs, colds, etc.
- It stimulates the circulation so that fresh nutrients and oxygen are brought to the cells and carbon dioxide and waste products are removed.
- It reduces high blood pressure.
- It relieves stress and tension.
- It combats insomnia.
- It reduces and relieves headaches.
- It improves concentration.
- It raises self-esteem and lifts depression.
- It reduces pain and tension in the muscles and joints.
- It improves mobility of the joints.
- It stimulates the sweat and sebaceous glands so that waste products are more rapidly eliminated and the skin is naturally moisturized. As the dead skin cells are removed, pores are encouraged to remain open, allowing increased skin respiration, suppleness and elasticity. Your skin looks healthy and glowing.
- It helps the digestion and absorption of food and encourages elimination thus preventing and alleviating constipation during the detox.
- It promotes the activity of the kidneys which enhances the elimination of waste products and reduces fluid retention.
- It helps menstrual problems such as PMT, period pains and irregular menstruation.
- It improves the efficiency of the respiratory system. Carbon dioxide is removed more efficiently and oxygen is absorbed more effectively. The breath will slow down and deepen.
- It promotes well-being.

Preparation for your massage

The time and place

Try to choose a time and place when you will not be disturbed. Take the phone off the hook, ensure that the room is warm and soften the lighting (you may wish to burn some candles). Play some soothing relaxation music to help you to create a peaceful space.

The massage oils

Your massage oil, also known as the carrier oil/base oil/fixed oil, should be a vegetable, nut or seed oil. It should also be cold pressed, unrefined and additive free. Such oils will have therapeutic properties and contain vitamins, minerals and fatty acids. I do not recommend mineral oil (purified, light petroleum oil) such as commercial baby oil which tends to clog the pores, is not easily absorbed and does not possess the nutritional value of vegetable, nut and seed oils. Mineral oil is used by the cosmetics industry because it does not become rancid but it remains on the skin like an 'oil slick' and prevents it from breathing.

Three of the most popular massage oils include:

- Sweet almond oil
  Extracted by cold pressing, sweet almond oil contains many vitamins, minerals and fatty acids. It is suitable for all types of skin, particularly dry, sensitive or prematurely aged skin. It is easily absorbed, does not have a strong odour and is a lovely light oil. You do not want your oil to be thick, heavy and sticky. Sweet almond oil was favoured by Napoleon's wife Josephine.

- Apricot kernel oil
  Apricot kernel is also suitable for all skin types and is a nourishing, enriching oil. It is similar to sweet almond oil but is more expensive as it is produced in smaller quantities.

- Sesame oil
  Sesame oil may be used for all types of skin. It is widely used in India in Ayurvedic medicine for its therapeutic effects. Do not use the strongly-flavoured dark brown oil with the nutty aroma which is used in Chinese cookery unless you want to smell like a restaurant all day! High quality suitable oil is available from aromatherapy suppliers (see Useful addresses).

If you want to, you can blend more than one carrier oil together to create your own special individual blend. Why not try adding one of the three following oils to your main oil?

- Jojoba
  A wonderful oil for the skin as it nourishes, moisturizes and penetrates deeply. Jojoba is very stable and therefore keeps well. It is a more expensive oil but well worth it.

- Evening primrose oil
  Evening primrose oil is widely used in capsule form as a nutritional supplement to treat conditions such as PMT, allergies (particularly skin and respiratory problems), heart disease, arthritis and even hyperactivity in children.

- Calendula oil
  Calendula oil is renowned for its anti-inflammatory, hormonal, healing and soothing properties. It is excellent for cracks and chapped hands and feet, irritated itchy red areas of the skin as well as broken veins and varicose veins.

You can add essential oils to your base oils to create your own detoxifying aromatherapy blend (see page 123 for details).

The sequence

Ideally, you should try to massage your complete body once a day to assist the detoxification process. If time is limited then instead of rushing your way through the whole sequence, concentrate on one or two areas, e.g. the legs and feet one day, your neck and shoulders the next. After a few days you will have massaged your entire body. You could select the areas according to your needs. For instance, if you want to work on your cellulite then make sure you carry out the leg massage daily. If you have a headache, perform the neck and shoulder and face and scalp routine. If you want to work on your constipation and improve the tone of your abdominal muscles then focus on the abdomen massage. You will need to apply a small amount of oil – all of the oil will be absorbed by the end of your treatment so there is no need to worry about feeling sticky.

Leg sequence
This sequence is great for stimulating the circulation, removing toxins, preventing varicose veins, reducing swelling and it will improve your cellulite.

Position for massage

Sit down on the floor or on a bed with one leg outstretched in front of you and the other leg bent with a foot flat on the ground. All the movements are performed up the leg towards the lymph glands in the groin to get rid of the toxins and poisonous substances.

1 Lower leg – firm stroking

Pour a small amount of oil onto the palm of one hand and rub your hands together to warm the oil. Stroke firmly up the bent leg from your heel to the back of your knee using the palms of one or both hands. Then stroke up the front of the leg too – you will not need so much pressure on the front of the lower leg as this is a bony area.

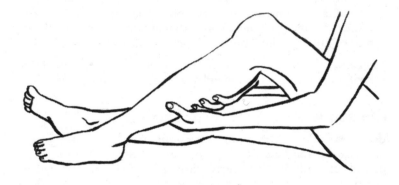

figure 3 lower leg – firm stroking

2 Calf muscles – decongesting

Still keeping your knee bent, place both hands flat down on your calf muscles. Use alternate hands to pick up, squeeze and release your calf muscles. These movements will remove any toxins that have accumulated in the deeper tissues, bring blood containing oxygen and nutrients to the area and prevent and relieve muscle spasms and stiffness.

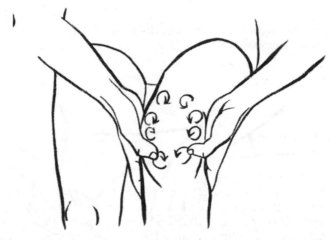

figure 4 calf muscles – decongesting

3 Knee – mobilizing
Place the pads of both thumbs just below the knee and use small circular movements all around your kneecap. These movements will help to improve and maintain mobility of your knees.

figure 5 knee – mobilizing

4 Thighs – detoxifying and cellulite busting
Use both hands to firmly stroke up the leg from the knee towards the lymph glands in the groin. Now use alternate hands to pick up, squeeze and release the inner, middle and outer thigh muscles. Notice how warm the area feels as you

work. These movements really help to break down any fatty deposits and if performed regularly can greatly improve the shape of your thighs.

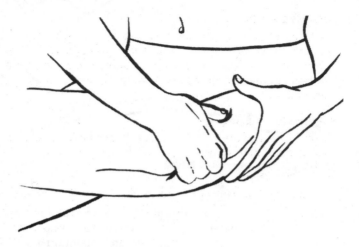

figure 6 thighs – detoxifying and cellulite busting

Finally, lightly clench your fists and bring them down in quick succession to pound your thighs.

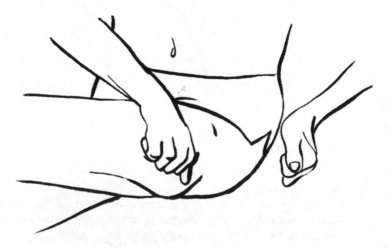

figure 7 thighs – toning

This will reduce the fatty deposits and give you beautifully-toned legs. Finish your leg routine with some stroking and then repeat on the other leg.

Foot sequence

Foot massage is not only relaxing but it will also help to improve the health of the whole body. According to reflexology, the feet are a mirror of the whole body and by massaging the feet you're assisting the detoxification of all the major organs of elimination.

Position for massage

Sit down on the floor, bed or chair. Bend the knee and place the foot to be treated on the opposite thigh.

1   Foot stroking
Using a small amount of oil, with one hand on the side of the foot and the other on the top stroke firmly up the foot several times.

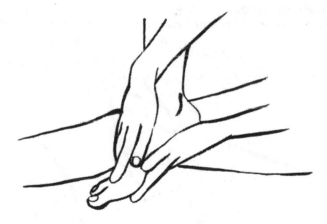

figure 8 foot stroking

2   Thumb circling
Use both thumbs to make small circular movements all over the sole of the foot. This loosens up the muscles and tendons and stimulates all the vital organs.

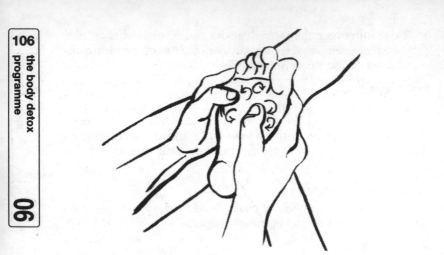

figure 9 thumb circling

3 Toe loosening
   Slowly stretch and circle each of your toes clockwise and
   anticlockwise. This not only loosens your toes but also
   stimulates the reflexology head zones, clearing out the
   sinuses, catarrh and mucus.

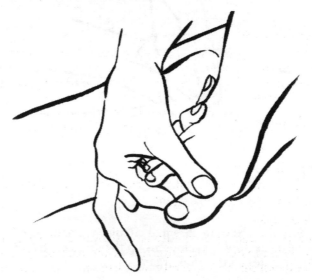

figure 10 toe loosening

4 Ankle loosening

Use your thumbs or fingertips to make circular movements all around the ankle joints. Then gently and slowly circle your ankle clockwise and anticlockwise. These movements encourage flexibility of the foot and reduce any fluid that has accumulated around the ankle. Repeat on the other foot.

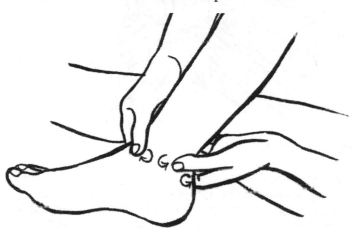

figure 11 ankle loosening

Neck and shoulder sequence

Neck and shoulder massage is excellent for relieving stress and tension and is wonderful for preventing and alleviating headaches. During the detox you should be avoiding painkillers. Instead of reaching for the paracetamol or aspirin try this instead. Over a period of time you will notice how much more freely your neck moves – reversing the car will be so much easier.

Position for massage

Sit on a chair with both feet flat on the ground or on the floor ensuring that your back is straight.

1 Neck stroking

Allow your head to drop forwards slightly and place your hands behind your neck, fingertips at the base of the skull. Stroke down the neck several times using the flat hands and feel the tension dissolving.

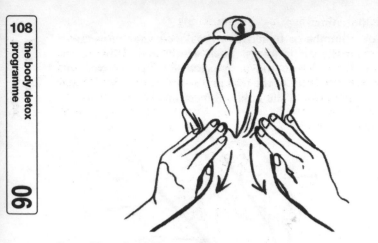

figure 12 neck stroking

2 Neck – loosening and detoxifying

Place the fingertips of one hand on the right hand side of the neck and the fingertips of the other hand on the left hand side of the neck. Perform small circular movements using your fingertips, working down the neck from top to bottom. Repeat several times. These movements help to break down knots, disperse toxins and improve mobility in the neck.

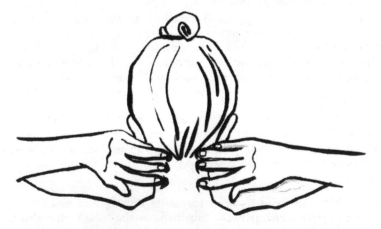

figure 13 neck loosening

3 Shoulders – decongesting and loosening

Reach across the front of your chest and place your right hand on your left shoulder and pick up and squeeze the muscles of the left shoulder. As you pick up, squeeze and release you are bringing the deeper toxins to the surface and releasing pent-up tension. Now massage across the top of your right shoulder by reaching across the front of your chest with your left hand.

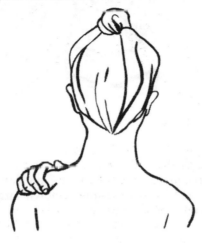

figure 14 shoulders – decongesting

Back sequence

This is a difficult area to reach but well worth it as most of us experience aches and pains in our lower back sometimes.

Position for massage

Sit on a stool or on the edge of a chair making sure that your feet are flat on the ground. If you are sitting on a chair you need to sit on the edge so that you can reach around to the back of your body. You can also stand up with your feet shoulder width apart.

1 Stroking the back

Place your hands behind your back, one flat palm either side of the spine. Stroke firmly down your back several times to bring increased blood flow to the area, relieve tension and flush out the toxins.

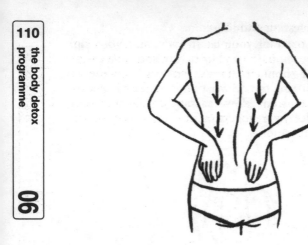

figure 15 stroking the back

2 Detoxifying the buttock area
   Place one flat palm at the top of each buttock and circle
   vigorously over the area to break down fatty deposits and
   decongest and tone the buttocks.

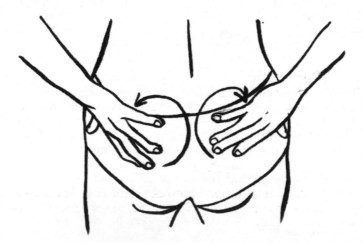

figure 16 detoxifying the buttock area

3 Loosening and decongesting the back
Place your thumbs onto the dimples (if you can find them) which are located at the base of your back either side of the spine. Perform small, deep circular movements, working up your back as far as you can. If you find any hard, knotty areas, circle over them as deeply as is comfortable with your thumbs. You can use your fingertips instead, if you find it easier.

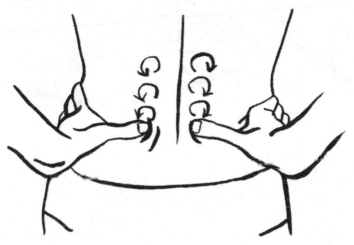

figure 17 loosening the back

Abdomen sequence

During the detox we want to encourage the bowels to move as freely as possible – two or three times a day would be ideal. This sequence will help you if you become constipated or bloated and will greatly assist the detoxification process.

Position for massage

The best position is laying on your back with your knees bent up to ensure complete relaxation of the abdominal muscles. You can also sit on a chair with your feet on the floor.

1 Stroking the abdomen
Place both hands, one on top of the other, on your navel. Make large slow circular movements working in a clockwise direction.

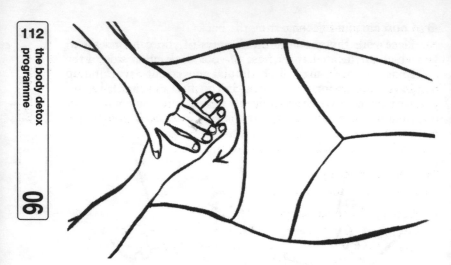

figure 18 stroking the abdomen

2 Stimulating the colon
   This technique is marvellous for constipation! Place your
   fingertips at the bottom right hand side of your abdomen
   and perform small circular movements working up the right
   hand side of the abdomen (ascending colon), across the
   abdomen area (transverse colon), then down the left hand
   side (descending colon). Finish with some stroking.

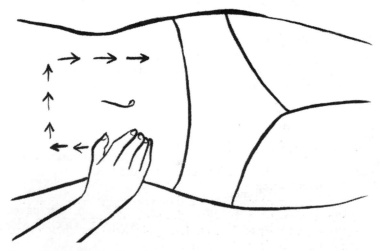

figure 19 stimulating the colon

Arm and hand sequence

Massage of the arms and hands is very beneficial for those of you who use them extensively in the course of your work, e.g. working at a computer. In addition, when you massage the hands you are treating all the organs, glands and structures of your body as according to hand reflexology, our health is mirrored in our hands (see *Teach Yourself Hand Reflexology* for more information). Massage of the arm and hand is also invaluable for reducing puffy wrists and arms.

Position for massage

Sit on a chair or on the floor.

1 Arm and hand stroking

Lift up your right arm to aid lymph drainage and stroke firmly up the arm from the wrist towards the lymph glands in the armpits.

figure 20 arm and hand stroking

2 Arm decongesting

Place the palm of your left hand on your right lower arm and make a V-shape with your thumb and fingers. Pick up, squeeze and release the muscles, again working up towards the lymph glands in the armpit.

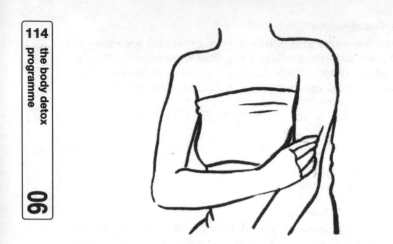

figure 21 arm decongesting

3 Wrist and hand detoxifying
With a loosely clenched fist work into the palm of your hand
using circular movements to loosen up the muscles, tendons
and joints. You are improving elimination of all the toxins
from the body. Use your thumb and fingertips to perform
small circular movements around the wrist and then interlock
your fingers and circle the wrist clockwise and anticlockwise.

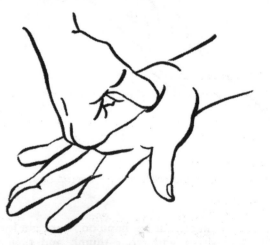

figure 22 wrist and hand detoxifying

4 Finger loosening

Use your thumb and index finger to gently stretch each finger and thumb and then circle each one individually. These movements will not only loosen the joints but will also decongest mucus and catarrh from the head area.

Repeat the arm and hand sequence on the other arm and hand.

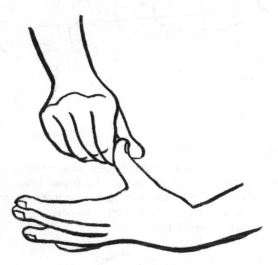

figure 23 finger loosening

Face and scalp sequence

A good face and scalp massage will drain away toxins, promote the regeneration of skin cells, release tension, stimulate hair growth, relieve headaches, restore mental clarity and concentration and make you look younger.

Position for massage

Sit on a chair or, if you prefer, relax on the bed.

1 Face stroking

Place both hands palms down on your forehead and fingertips facing each other. Stroke across your forehead, across your cheeks and then across your chin.

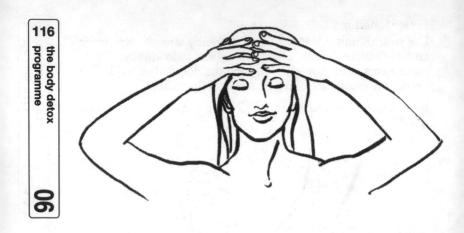

figure 24 face stroking

2 Eyebrows and eyes
   To tone the eyebrows, gently use your thumb and index
   finger to lightly squeeze along the brow bone. To relieve
   puffiness and to prevent and reduce fine lines, use your index
   finger or index and middle fingers to perform small circular
   movements around each eye.

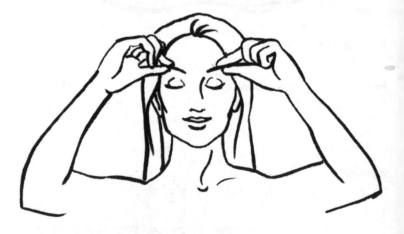

figure 25 eyebrows – toning

3 Massaging the ears
Use your thumbs and forefingers to gently and slowly massage your ears.

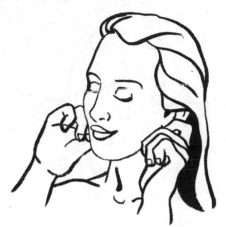

figure 26 massaging the ears

4 Releasing jaw tension
Use your thumbs and index fingers to gently squeeze and release the jawbone.

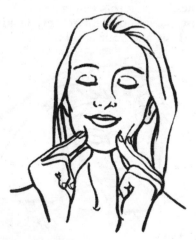

figure 27 releasing jaw tension

5 Mouth
Using your fingertips, gently circle all around your mouth to help to prevent wrinkles from appearing.

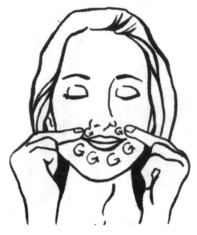

figure 28 mouth

6 Scalp loosening and detoxifying
Place the pads of the fingers of both hands on top of your head and perform small circular movements all over your entire scalp. These movements will increase circulation to the scalp and assist the removal of toxins, making your hair healthy and lustrous and your mind clear.

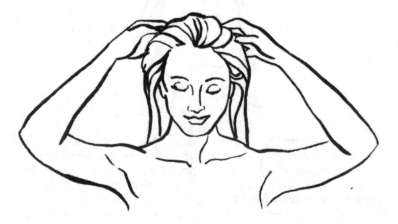

figure 29 scalp loosening

7 Face and scalp toning
Use the pads of your fingertips to tap very lightly all over your face and scalp. This will tone the muscles and make you feel energized and revitalized.

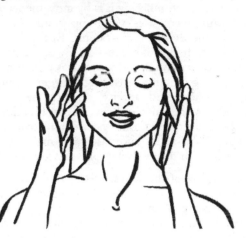

figure 30 face and scalp toning

If you enjoy self-massage you may be inspired to massage your family and friends. Why not try my *Teach Yourself Massage* book in this series?

Exercise

'Eating properly will not by itself keep well a person who does not exercise, for food and exercise, being opposite in effect, work together to produce perfect health.'

Hippocrates

Exercise is vital to good health and will enable you to enhance the detoxification process as well as keep you fit and supple. Exercise is an excellent way to stimulate the intestines and get the bowels moving. During exercise, the diaphragm and abdominal muscles work in such a way that the intestines are squeezed and kneaded and are stimulated into action. Those who lead a sedentary life can suffer from weak abdominal muscles that are lacking in tone and are incapable of supporting the intestines in their correct place. Individuals who lead an active life and are employed in occupations that involve plenty of moving around rarely suffer from constipation, provided that they eat the right foods and drink enough water. Exercise is also vital for the efficient functioning of the lymphatic system. Unlike the heart-driven circulatory system, the lymphatic system has no central pump in it. One of the ways of stimulating it is by movements of the body's muscles and thus exercise is very important for the efficient functioning of the lymphatic system. Regular exercise also improves elimination through the skin by stimulating sweating and helping detoxification. In addition, it is a key to maintaining and improving lung function, ensuring a larger supply of oxygen which brings strength and vitality, an increase in energy, and clears the mind. Exercise also improves heart function, stimulates circulation, boosts the immune system, improves flexibility of joints, eases muscular aches and pains and makes you feel more equipped to deal with the everyday pressures of life.

These are just a few of the ways that exercise will enhance the organs of elimination. It is not necessary to spend vast amounts of money joining a gym or going to exercise classes every day. You just need to clear a space in your lounge or bedroom or get out into the fresh air.

A little exercise (i.e. 20 minutes) a day is far better than a two-hour workout once a week. Little and often is the golden rule. It is really easy to introduce a small amount of exercise into your daily routine. In this way, you will not have any excuse to give up and you will not get too tired and put off by exercise. The benefits that you will derive after just a few days will give you the inspiration to carry on!

Easy ways to exercise:

- A 20-minute walk daily is an excellent way to exercise. Do it first thing in the morning and then you don't have to spend all day thinking about it and making excuses as to why you shouldn't do it!
- If you work and have difficulty incorporating a daily walk into your routine, then try to go for a walk in your lunch hour, especially if there is a nice park nearby.
- You can also walk up and down the stairs for about five to ten minutes, which will really stimulate your abdominal muscles.
- Try to stop using escalators and lifts and walk up and down the stairs instead.
- Walk on the spot for five minutes and then jog on the spot for five minutes.

- If possible walk the children to school instead of taking the car. They will probably complain at first but they will derive benefit too.
- Invest in a skipping rope and skip for five minutes each day.
- If you like to go to exercise classes then I would strongly recommend a yoga or tai chi class.

Breathing

Breathing is another key part of a detox regime. If you learn how to breathe properly you will speed up the elimination of toxins through your lungs. Most of us breathe very shallowly and therefore do not use the lungs to their full capacity. In fact, the majority of us only use the top quarter to one third of the lungs!

Expansion of the lungs and diaphragm massages the organs of the abdomen including the liver and promotes the circulation of oxygen. This increase in oxygen enables our cells, tissues and organs to work far more efficiently. As you breathe out you exhale carbon dioxide which must be expelled to prevent the build-up of toxins. Deep breathing also brings benefits on a psychological level. It is the most wonderful nerve tonic. Think of when you are feeling anxious how shallow and fast your breathing is. If you breathe deeply and correctly you will feel peaceful, calm and more able to cope.

The following exercise will take you just a few minutes every day and I can assure you that once you have experienced the benefits of oxygen, the elixir of life, you will want to continue this exercise after the detox.

The full breath-of-life detox exercise

Position for breathing

To carry out this exercise either lie down comfortably or, if you prefer, sit up. If you can lie down you will probably find this exercise most relaxing. You can do this exercise in bed, particularly if you have trouble sleeping or if your mind is full of persistent thoughts that are difficult to switch off.

If you decide to sit up do make sure that your back is straight. You can sit on a chair with your feet flat on the ground or on the floor supported by pillows if required. Make sure you wear loose-fitting clothes so that your breathing is not restricted.

1 Place one hand on the abdomen and one on your chest.
2 Take a slow deep breath through your nose and as you inhale feel the hand on your abdomen rise. The hand on the chest should not move. As you breathe in, try to count to four. If you can only make it to three do not worry.
3 Hold your deep breath of four counts (if you can).
4 Now exhale very slowly through your mouth to the count of eight and feel your abdomen collapsing under your hand. As you breathe out feel yourself expelling all the poisonous toxins. Breathe in for four – hold for four – exhale for eight.
5 Practice this deep breathing for a few minutes daily. If you feel proficient, try to take the exercises further.

More advanced breathing exercise

1 Stay in the same position with one hand on the abdomen and one on the chest.
2 Inhale deeply, feeling the hand on your abdomen rise and when you feel it cannot expand any further take in some more air and feel the chest expand too. This process (i.e. abdomen expand – chest expand) should take about eight counts.
3 Exhale slowly, allowing the air to release from the chest first and then the abdomen. You should aim to make your exhalation eight counts too. Inhale for eight (abdomen then chest) – exhale for 8 (chest then abdomen). Practise this deep-breathing exercise for a few minutes daily. In time you will no longer find it necessary to place the hands on the chest and abdomen.

Enhancing the body detox

Aromatherapy detox

Aromatherapy is the use of essential oils in treatments to strive for physical, mental and spiritual health equilibrium. It is a very powerful therapy and if you find this brief section interesting, you may wish to read my *Teach Yourself Aromatherapy* book in this series.

The healing properties of essential oils have been harnessed for centuries and some oils are particularly effective for enhancing the detoxification process. There are a whole host of ways of using these precious essences but for the purposes of the body detox I will explain how to use them in your daily bath/shower and in your daily self-massage routine.

Detoxifying baths

Essential oils may be used on their own or may be added to your Epsom salts bath.

Method

1 Fill up the bath and then scatter six drops of essential oil into the water. Do not add the essential oil(s) until you have run the bath completely otherwise the oil will evaporate and you will lose the therapeutic properties before you climb in!
2 Disperse the oil thoroughly. If you inadvertently sit down on six drops of neat essential oil you will jump up very quickly again.
3 Stay in the bath for about 15 minutes to enjoy the therapeutic effects of the oils.

Detoxifying showers

If you do not have a bath or you are pushed for time then opt for an aromatherapy shower. Simply sprinkle your six drops of essential oil onto a sponge or flannel and gently rub all over your body towards the end of your shower. Then continue your shower as usual.

Alternatively, if you wish, you can add your six drops of essential oil to two teaspoons of the carrier oil you are using for your massage and apply it to your body before you step into the shower.

Detoxifying aromamassage

To enhance your self-massage why not add a detoxifying essential oil to your massage oil? The combination of pure essential oils and massage is a very potent tool for purification. You must never use essential oils in an undiluted form as they are highly concentrated and may irritate the skin.

To make your aromatherapy detox, blend three drops of essential oil to two teaspoons of carrier oil. You do not need to add more than three drops as an increased concentration of essential oil does not imply that the formula will be more effective. Excessive amounts of essential oil can create unpleasant side effects and reactions. After you have blended your detox formula, rub a small amount onto the back of your hand. If you like the smell it will do you good!

Detoxifying oils for the body

Essential oils possess many therapeutic effects. I will focus on a handful of essential oils which will assist the organs of elimination and relieve some of the side effects encountered during a detox.

To stimulate the circulation
- Black pepper
- Eucalyptus
- Ginger
- Lemon
- Lemongrass
- Rosemary.

To dexoify the lymphatic system
- Carrot seed
- Cedarwood
- Cypress
- Fennel
- Grapefruit
- Lemon
- Lime
- Mandarin
- Rosemary.

To boost the immune system
- Carrot seed
- Lavender
- Lemon
- Lemongrass
- Mandarin
- Tea tree
- Thyme.

To combat constipation
- Black pepper
- Carrot seed
- Fennel

- Ginger
- Marjoram
- Rosemary
- Thyme.

To relieve diarrhoea
- Black pepper
- Camomile
- Ginger
- Peppermint
- Rosemary.

To alleviate flatulence
- Camomile
- Fennel
- Ginger
- Marjoram
- Peppermint
- Rosemary.

To combat indigestion
- Basil
- Fennel
- Ginger
- Lemon
- Peppermint.

To eliminate cellulite
- Cypress
- Fennel
- Grapefruit
- Juniper
- Lemon
- Rosemary.

To reduce fluid
- Cypress
- Fennel
- Geranium
- Juniper
- Lemon
- Rosemary.

To stimulate the lungs

- Basil
- Cajeput
- Eucalyptus
- Frankincense
- Rosemary.

I could easily have selected more than 20 essential oils in each section but for the sake of simplicity I have listed just a few of the most useful oils. You may notice that some essential oils appear very frequently on the lists. If I had to choose my top six detoxifying oils they would be:

- Black pepper
- Fennel
- Grapefruit
- Juniper
- Lemon
- Rosemary.

Why not start off by buying two or three of these oils and if you enjoy using them, gradually add to your collection? For suppliers of high-quality pure essential oils please refer to the Useful Addresses.

Hand reflexology detox

Hand reflexology is a simple, natural method of applying gentle pressure to the hands, which can be seen as a mirror image of the body. All of the structures and organs are reflected in the hands. By using hand reflexology in the detox we can release the impurities and toxins that are impairing the functioning of our bodies.

Reflexology is more commonly performed on the feet but the reflex points on the hands are so much easier to reach and you can treat yourself at any time and in any place. No one will even be aware that you are doing anything!

I will not be describing all the reflex points in this book (see *Teach Yourself Hand Reflexology* for complete details); we will learn some of the main detoxification points.

Hand reflex detox routine

This simple routine will take less than five minutes (longer at first perhaps whilst you familiarize yourself with the routine). You can practise it anywhere but if you really want to relax, get yourself comfortable in your favourite chair or sit on the sofa. Place a cushion or pillow on your lap, rest your hand on it and off you go!

There are many techniques used in reflexology but the only one you need to learn for this routine is 'caterpillar walking'. The outer edge of the thumb is used for this technique. If you are unsure about which is the inner and which is the outer edge of your thumb, place your hand palm downwards onto a flat surface such as a table. The tip of your thumb that is touching the surface is the outer edge and this will be the working area of your thumb. Practise caterpillar walking on your forearm.

To caterpillar walk, bend the first joint of your thumb just slightly and then unbend the joint slightly. Notice that you have moved forward a little. Repeat this movement to walk right the way up your forearm. As you reach your elbow, turn your hand round and walk from your elbow to your wrist. Practise on your other forearm so that you can caterpillar walk with both thumbs. Ensure that you are always moving forwards, as the thumb walking technique is never performed backwards or sideways. Check that your thumb is only slightly bent – it should be neither too bent nor too straight. If your thumb is too

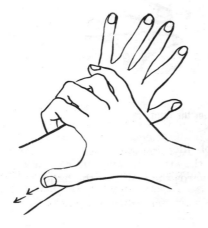

figure 31 caterpillar walking on the forearm

bent you will dig your nail into your hand. It is only the first joint of the thumb that moves – the second joint of the thumb does not move but helps to create leverage. Although the entire hand participates in this movement the first joint of the thumb is the only moving part.

After performing caterpillar walking on your forearm, practise it on the palm of your hand.

Left hand

1 Upper lymphatics – location: webbing between the fingers. With your right thumb and index finger gently squeeze the webbing between each of the fingers. Repeat several times.

2 Left lung – location: upper third of the palm of the hand. With your right thumb, caterpillar walk across the hand in horizontal rows covering the upper third of the palm of the hand. You will need to do three or four rows.

Now turn your hand over and use your index and middle fingers to finger walk down the upper third of the top of the hand, starting at the base of the fingers.

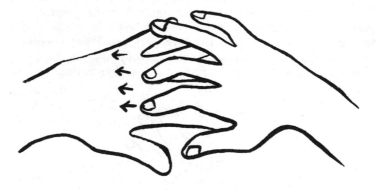

figure 32 walking over the lung area

3 Left kidney/bladder – location: on the palm below the webbing of the thumb and index finger, continuing diagonally towards the inside of the hand.

Place your right thumb, pointing downwards, just below the webbing of the thumb and index finger and circle lightly over this area. Walk diagonally towards the inside of the hand towards the bladder and gently circle your thumb over it a few times.

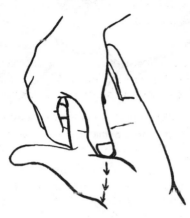

figure 33 working from the kidney down towards the bladder

4 Intestines – location: lower third of the palm of the hand. Caterpillar walk across the lower third of the palm of the hand. It should take you three or four rows.

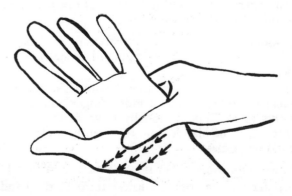

figure 34 caterpillar walking over the intestines

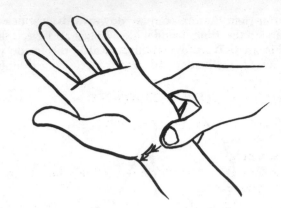

figure 35 treating the lymph nodes of the groin

5 Lymph nodes of the groin — location: circles the wrist.
   Use your right thumb to walk all the way round the wrist
   both front and back.

Right hand

1 Upper lymphatics – location: webbing between the fingers.
   With your left thumb and index finger gently squeeze the
   webbing between each of the fingers. Repeat several times.

2 Right lung – location: upper third of the palm of the hand.
   Use your left thumb to caterpillar walk from the little finger
   side right across the hand in horizontal rows. You will need
   to do three to four rows.

3 Right kidney/bladder – location: between the webbing of the
   thumb and index finger, continuing diagonally towards the
   inside of the hand.
   Place your left thumb, pointing downwards, just below the
   webbing of the thumb and index finger and lightly circle
   over this area. Walk diagonally towards the inside of the
   hand towards the bladder and then gently circle your thumb
   over it a few times.

4 Intestines – location: lower third of the palm of the hand.
   Caterpillar walk across the lower third of the hand using
   about three or four rows.

5 Lymph nodes of the groin – location: circles the wrist.
   Use your left thumb to walk all the way round the wrist both
   front and back.

Whilst you are on your detox you may find that some of the points feel slightly sensitive. This is to be expected, as your organs of elimination will be working hard.

Your body detox summary

- Dry skin brushing (less than five minutes)
- Hot/Cold shower
- Tongue scraping
- Self-massage – if time available whole body but if not focus on one or two areas
- Exercise – 20 minutes daily
- Breathing – a few minutes daily
- Epsom salts bath – every three to four days.

Optional:

- Aromatherapy detox – add essential oils to your daily bath/shower and/or blend a detox formula for your self-massage
- Hand reflexology detox (less than five minutes).

21-day body detox checklist

		1	2	3	4	5	6	7	8	9	10	11	12	13	14	15	16	17	18	19	20	21
Dry skin brushing																						
Hot/Cold shower																						
Tongue scraping																						
Self-massage																						
Exercise																						
Breathing																						
Epsom salts bath every 3–4 days																						
Aromatherapy oils	O P T I O N A L																					
Hand reflexology																						

Why not complete this body detox checklist to see if you are keeping to the guidelines? Just tick the boxes as you did with the daily food checklist (page 92).

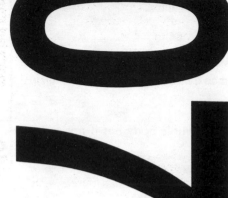

07

the mind and spirit detox programme

In this chapter you will learn:
- about various techniques for detoxing the mind
- how best to detox the spirit.

Up until now we have concentrated on ways of detoxifying the body, yet the connection between body, mind and spirit has long been recognized. Now we need to focus on cleansing the mind and spirit if our detox is to be completely successful. It is essential to look at every aspect of our life if we are to totally transform ourselves. For a completely successful detox we must focus on cleansing the mind and the spirit. It is not only your body that needs cleansing and nourishing – your mind and spirit yearns for purification too!

Detox the mind

There is no point in having a wonderfully cleansed body if our minds are full of negative thought patterns and cluttered with emotions such as fear, anger, hatred and jealousy.

Our thoughts and feelings can have a deep impact on our health. Stress-related hormones can actually weaken our immune systems, raise our blood pressure and upset our digestion – indeed any of our systems can become out of balance and the result is disease.

Negative thoughts are extremely detrimental to our health and well-being. Negative thoughts attract negative influences whereas positive thoughts attract positive influences. Emotions such as fear and panic not only encourage disease but also intensify any underlying illness.

Positive emotions such as love, hope and happiness can interrupt these negative emotions. They can exert a protective effect against fear, anger, worry and despair, which lead to disease. Positive emotions can be seen as 'blockers' and they have the ability to drive out the negative. It is not possible to entertain a positive emotion and a negative emotion – you cannot laugh and be very angry at the same time. The laughter can replace the anger. Think of when you are having an argument – if laughter is brought into the equation the anger soon dissipates and you realize how silly your anger was in the first place.

It is difficult to prevent ourselves from becoming overwhelmed with our worries and fears and the majority of us can feel down sometimes. If we allow our mind to continue in this way we are unable to think straight and plan and we can even become very depressed and then we are unable to function at all. It seems as if there is no way out!

A mind detox will enable you to clear away these negative thoughts and toxic feelings and make space for a new positive you!

Do you need a mind detox?

Try out this questionnaire to reveal if your mind needs a detox.

- Do you feel stressed and anxious?
- Do you feel tired and fatigued?
- Do you lay awake at night with racing thoughts?
- Do you find it difficult to think straight and stay focused?
- Do you have difficulty in getting out of bed?
- Do you feel discontented and/or depressed?
- Do you feel angry and resentful?
- Do you feel stuck in a dead-end job?
- Are your relationships unfulfilling?
- Do you spend time worrying?
- Do you feel bored?
- Do you think the cup is half empty, rather than half full?
- Do you feel lacking in confidence and self-esteem?
- Do you lack creativity?

If you have answered yes to any of these questions then your mind is in need of a detox! So let us now look at ways of detoxing your mind.

Affirmations

During the detox programme (and indeed afterwards) when you are feeling low, vulnerable, unmotivated and things are not going your way, a few positive affirmations will set you on the right track!

Affirmations are a way of changing the way that you think. They will enable you to think positively and to feel good about yourself. Affirmations are short positive statements which are repeated. In this way the subconscious mind can be retrained so that negative thoughts can be eliminated or at least reduced. They are based on the idea that if you tell yourself something often enough you will believe it and it will become true.

Affirmations can be said (or thought) anywhere and at any time. Say them to yourself at least five times. You can sit yourself down quietly at some point in your day or if you prefer they can be said whilst you are on the move. Repeat them to yourself whilst you are looking in the mirror brushing your hair or on your way to work while stuck at the traffic lights. As the day progresses and you encounter new challenges you can repeat your affirmations or invent new ones appropriate to the situation! Before you go to sleep create an affirmation and notice how much more positive you feel the next day. It is not necessary to say an affirmation out loud although it is thought to be more powerful. You can think an affirmation to yourself or you can even write it down and stick the piece of paper, for instance, on the fridge in the kitchen.

Affirmations:

- Can be said out loud
- Can be thought
- Can be written down
- Should be said at least five times (if you still feel negative, repeat your affirmations five more times)
- Should be positive
- Should be brief
- Should be said with meaning
- Should be believed in.

Examples of affirmations:

- 'I am happy.'
- 'I am healthy.'
- 'I am beautiful.'
- 'I am loved.'
- 'I believe in myself.'
- 'I am peaceful and calm.'
- 'I am relaxed.'
- 'My mind is clear.'
- 'I am content.'
- 'I am confident.'
- 'I will succeed.'
- 'I am brilliant.'

If you repeat your affirmations often enough you will really start to believe in yourself. As you feel positive about yourself you will generate positivity all around you. Your self-esteem and confidence will be boosted so that if you are criticized you will not be so affected by it.

Once you feel in a positive frame of mind try to compliment a friend, colleague or even stranger. The compliment, of course, must be genuine but there is always at least one good thing that you can say about everyone you meet; if you make a friend's day this will in turn make you feel even more positive!

Breathing

The breathing exercises described on pages 121–2 as part of the body detox are also invaluable for de-stressing and detoxing the mind. This will still the mind so that you are relaxed yet focused and alert and prepared to deal with the stresses and strains of the day.

Practise the full breath-of-life detox and as you inhale feel as if you are breathing in positivity and energy. As you exhale imagine that you are expelling and letting go of all your negativity and worries. Repeat for as long as you feel necessary to rid yourself of your mental clutter.

Bach flower remedies

Bach flower remedies are an excellent detox tool since they help to dissolve blockages such as negative emotions thus enabling us to feel positive and able to cope with problems that confront us in our everyday life.

Bach flower remedies were created by the physician Dr Edward Bach who became disillusioned with the orthodox idea of treating symptoms with medicines that often had harmful side effects. His system of healing is intended to treat the person and deal with the root cause of the problem rather than treating the disease. He firmly believed in the philosophy that a healthy mind ensures a healthy body.

Dr Bach discovered 38 flowers which cover the many negative states from which we all can suffer. It is well known that persistent worry lowers the body's vitality and its natural resistance to disease so that physical conditions are allowed to develop. By treating a negative state of mind we are restoring balance to the body by eliminating the physical problems resulting from an unbalanced mind.

The remedies are completely natural, safe, non-habit forming and have no harmful side effects. They may be taken alongside other medications with no risk of conflict and it is impossible to overdose on them.

You may take a single Bach flower remedy or a combination of remedies. To prepare a remedy fill a 30 ml dropper bottle with pure spring water, add a teaspoon of brandy for preservation purposes and add two drops of your chosen remedy. You may use more than one remedy at once but I usually try not to use more than three. People often ask how long the remedies take to work. It depends on how long your mind has been toxic! Negative thoughts and emotions that have developed recently should pass away quickly whereas deep-rooted problems will take longer before they heal.

I have listed below my top seven flower essences which I consider to be most appropriate for a detox:

Crab apple

Crab apple cleanses both mind and body. Dr Bach described it as 'the remedy which helps us to get rid of anything we do not like either in our minds or bodies'. It will not only cleanse the mind of anything you do not like about yourself but it will also accelerate the elimination of toxins from the body.

Olive

During a detox, particularly in the first few days, it is a common reaction to feel tired. This normally happens when a dietary change is made. Olive is an excellent remedy for relieving tiredness and fatigue.

Walnut

This remedy is the 'link breaker' since it helps to break our negative cycles such as food addictions and entrenched thought patterns. It helps us to move forward and assists us with the necessary changes that we need to make during the detox.

White chestnut

This remedy is for persistent unwanted thoughts that go round and round in the mind. It is particularly useful not only if you are a worrier but also if you find it difficult to switch off your mind during the breathing and/or meditation sessions.

Hornbeam

Hornbeam is used for the 'Monday morning' feeling. It is ideal for those days when you feel apathetic and lethargic. Take your hornbeam and you will be able to face those cold showers and the hot water with lemon in!

Impatiens

This remedy is useful for anger, irritability, mood swings and a tendency to overreact. Particularly at the beginning of a detox you may be short tempered and agitated as you have given up caffeine and sugary foods which do not let go of you easily.

Honeysuckle

Honeysuckle is for those who cling on to the past. During a detox it is effective for those who think back to their former dietary habits and old ways. Honeysuckle helps you to stay in the present and adhere to your current eating regime.

Aromatherapy – essential oils to detox the mind

I have already described how aromatherapy oils can be used to enhance your body detox programme and details of how to prepare aromatherapy baths and aromamassage oils can be found on pages 122–6.

Essential oils, however, are not used exclusively for detoxification of the body. The inhalation of essential oils has a profound effect on the mind. It can help to dispel negative emotions such as fear, anger, grief, panic and obsessions. Essential oils also have the ability to induce positive emotions such as courage, confidence and strength. Three simple inhalation methods are described below:

Vaporizer

Essential oil burners are widely available and inexpensive. They are usually earthenware and are heated by a nightlight candle. Put a few teaspoons of water into the bowl on top and sprinkle approximately six drops of essential oil into the water. Then light the nightlight and as the water evaporates the room will become permeated with the aroma. Make sure that you keep the water topped up in the bowl and try to choose an oil burner with a deep reservoir.

Handkerchief/Tissue

Simply sprinkle a few drops of essential oil onto a handkerchief or tissue or even a cotton-wool ball held close to the nose and take a few deep breaths. You can then place the handkerchief in your pocket and then you can continue to inhale the aroma throughout the day as required.

Pillow

Sprinkle a few drops of essential oil onto your pillow for relief from problems such as insomnia. If desired, you could put the drops onto a piece of cotton wool and place it inside the pillowcase.

Essential oils to detox the mind

Condition	Aromatherapy oils
Addictions	Clary sage
Anger	Chamomile, cypress, ylang ylang
Apathy and lethargy	Ginger, lemongrass, lime, rosemary
Change	Cypress, frankincense
Concentration	Basil, lemon, rosemary
Confidence	Ginger, jasmine
Courage	Black pepper, fennel, ginger
Decision making	Basil, carrot seed
Depression	Bergamot, geranium, grapefruit, jasmine, lime, mandarin, rose, ylang ylang
Fear	Clary sage, jasmine, lavender, neroli, frankincense, ylang ylang
Grief	Cypress, frankincense, mandarin, marjoram, neroli, rose
Memory	Basil, black pepper, ginger, rosemary
Mental fatigue	Basil, peppermint, rosemary
Negativity	Jasmine, juniper, lime, mandarin
Resentment	Grapefruit, lemon
Stress and tension	Cedarwood, clary sage, cypress, geranium, grapefruit, mandarin, marjoram, neroli, patchouli, petitgrain, rose, sandalwood

Why not experiment with one or two essential oils to detox your mind?

Detox the spirit

The majority of people are aware of their physical and mental well-being! However, many choose to ignore the importance of their spiritual well-being or are simply unaware of it. When one is balanced on a spiritual level one is aware of one's inner self and exudes a very deep sense of peace and tranquillity. Many of us do not make the time or effort to connect with our true inner selves. We become so busy with our hectic lifestyles that we do not endeavour to take the time to be alone, to reflect, to meditate or to evolve our spirituality. It is vital not just to focus on the body and mind but on our spiritual health equilibrium too.

The chakras

It may seem ridiculous to you but we are not just a physical body. We are surrounded by subtle energy bodies that make up our 'aura' which varies enormously in size from one person to another. As well as the aura we also have energy centres known as 'chakras' (the word 'chakra' is a Sanskrit word meaning 'wheel', 'disc' or 'circle'). If these constantly revolving wheels of energy become unbalanced then disharmony and disease will result. We will take a brief look at the seven major chakras:

Base/root chakra
Colour: red.

Position: base of the spine between the anus and genitals.

The root chakra connects us with the physical world, i.e. the earth. If it is out of balance, we do not feel properly grounded. We may feel a sense of 'spaciness' or insecurity.

Sacral/abdomen chakra
Colour: orange.

Position: lower abdomen.

The sacral centre is connected with our sexuality and creativity. An imbalance can lead to problems with our sexual organs and relationships.

Solar plexus chakra
Colour: yellow.

Position: between the navel and the solar plexus.

If the solar plexus is out of balance we may experience low self-esteem, mood swings, an inability to relax as well as addictions.

Heart chakra

Colour: green and pink.

Position: centre of the chest.

Imbalances include an inability to love oneself and others unconditionally, depression and a lack of forgiveness.

Throat chakra

Colour: blue.

Position: throat.

An imbalance in the throat centre may lead to an inability to express one's feelings and ideas and creativity is blocked.

Third eye chakra

Colour: indigo.

Position: centre of the forehead.

If the third eye chakra is blocked our intuition is blocked and we lack inner wisdom.

Crown chakra

Colour: violet.

Position: top of the head.

This is our centre of spirituality and if it is out of balance we are unable or fearful of opening up to spiritual levels.

It is not only your body and mind that need a detox, your chakras need to be cleansed too. You will find that if you cleanse your chakras regularly you will feel totally at one with yourself.

Cleansing the chakras

1 Ensure that you are wearing loose-fitting clothes and sit in a comfortable position. Either sit cross-legged on the floor on several cushions or sit on a chair with your back straight with your feet touching the ground. This will help you to establish a strong connection to the earth so that you feel grounded and secure. Visualize roots coming out the soles of your feet (if you are sitting on a chair) or if you are sitting cross-legged imagine the roots emanating from the base of your spine.

2 Become aware of your breathing and practise your full breath-of-life exercise – breathe in for four counts – hold the breath for four – exhale for four. Repeat this breathing until your mind has released its mental clutter.

3 Turn your attention to your root chakra at the base of your spine and imagine that it is spinning and full of light. If it feels blocked or dull, imagine a whirlpool of light cleansing it and see it healthy and glowing with energy.

4 Now focus your attention slightly higher up on the sacral chakra just below the navel. Cleanse the chakra and visualize it glowing with health and energy.

5 Continue to cleanse each chakra in turn – the solar plexus chakra (above the navel), the heart chakra (in the centre of the chest), the throat chakra (in the throat), the third eye chakra (in the centre of the forehead) and the crown chakra (on the top of the head).

6 Once you have cleansed all the chakras bring your attention back to your breathing. Become aware of your contact with the ground and gently move your fingers and toes. Open your eyes very slowly.

NB If you find it difficult to visualize then you can hold your hands in front of each of the chakras as you perform this cleansing exercise.

At the end of this exercise if you have experienced any strange sensations or you felt that any of your chakras seemed to be blocked then make a note of it in your detox diary. Never be dismissive of any experiences you may have.

Meditation

Meditation is practised all over the world to detox the mind and spirit. It can help you to develop a sense of inner peace and evolve your spirituality.

It is very rare for someone to be able to drift into a deep meditative state when trying for the first time. The mind likes to wander. It usually takes some perseverance but be patient as it is wonderful to be able to empty your mind and reach deep within yourself to discover your true inner self.

1 Begin by finding a peaceful place and a time when you won't be disturbed. This may be under a tree, in your garden or in your lounge or bedroom. To create a meditative atmosphere,

light a candle or burn some aromatherapy oils to help you to relax.

2 Put yourself in a comfortable position. You may sit cross-legged on the floor on some pillows or upright on a chair with your feet flat on the ground. You may also lie down on the floor with cushions/pillows under your head and knees. During meditation you may become chilly so wrap a blanket around you or if you are lying down, cover yourself up with a blanket or towel. Once you are comfortable become aware of a strong connection with the earth and imagine that you have roots extending deep down into the centre of the earth.

3 Close your eyes and take a few deep breaths. Imagine you are inhaling healing white light and that this white light is absorbing any negative energy. As you exhale feel yourself releasing this energy. Repeat this breathing exercise noticing how relaxed and free from tension you feel.

4 Try to stay focused on the breath. If thoughts pop into your head then simply acknowledge them and stay focused on your breathing. Remain in this meditative state for just a few minutes at first and try to gradually build up to 20 minutes a day.

5 When you are ready to return, bring your awareness to your body, gently moving your fingers and toes. Slowly open your eyes and carry the deep sense of peace that has enveloped your body, mind and spirit with you throughout the day.

Aromatherapy – essential oils to detox the spirit

The healing power of aromatherapy can also be harnessed to detox the spirit (and aromatherapy is also excellent for cleansing and balancing the chakras). Essential oils provide an excellent aid to meditation when used in an essential oil burner (see page 138 for details). They may also be used in your bath/shower or added to your massage oil to create an aromatherapy blend.

Essential oils to detox the spirit

- Angelica seed – opens up the intuition and links us with our higher self. Useful for the brow and crown chakras.
- Benzoin – earths and grounds us and therefore detoxifies and balances the base chakra.

- Black pepper – cleanses the throat chakra thus encouraging creativity and communication.
- Carrot seed – unblocks the third eye chakra bestowing clarity and insight.
- Cedarwood – releases spiritual and emotional blockages that impede our development.
- Chamomile – brings peace to a troubled spirit. It purifies the solar plexus chakra.
- Clary sage – dispels the fear of opening up to our spirituality.
- Elemi – encourages stillness, peace and tranquillity. Elemi detoxifies the solar plexus and heart chakras.
- Fennel – cleanses the spirit of toxins and gives us the strength to face difficult situations.
- Frankincense – melts away blockages and moves us along our spiritual pathway enabling us to achieve a heightened state of spiritual awareness.
- Grapefruit – unblocks and transmutes negativity. Grapefruit helps us to restore our inner light.
- Hyssop – cleanses and purifies all the chakras. Hyssop is particularly indicated if there is a history of traumatic events.
- Jasmine – purifies the sacral chakra and balances and heals the solar plexus and heart centres.
- Lavender – helps to repair damage to the aura.
- Lemon – cleanses the spirit and fills us with renewed strength.
- Mandarin – gently detoxifies and heals the heart chakra.
- Myrrh – heals a deeply wounded soul and detoxifies the throat centre encouraging us to speak the truth.
- Neroli – fills the spirit with light.
- Patchouli – helps to establish a strong connection to the earth, promoting security.
- Pine – cleanses the chakras and drives out negativity.
- Rose – deeply cleanses the heart chakra filling us with love and compassion and dispelling sorrow and resentment.
- Rosemary – detoxifies the chakras, clears away confusion and sheds light on our purpose on this earth.
- Sage – purifies the aura of unwanted thoughts, cleanses the chakras and provides protection.
- Vetivert – detoxifies the chakras and is perfect for those who feel spiritually ungrounded.
- Ylang ylang – brings a wandering mind into a meditative state. Ylang ylang also detoxifies the heart and sacral centres.

Crystals

The healing powers of crystals have been recognized throughout the ages. Crystals can help to heal body, mind and spirit, enhance meditative powers, connect us with our spirituality, protect us against unwanted energies and to transform negative into positive energy.

One can work with large, small, uncut, polished, clear or coloured crystals. If a crystal is meant for you then you will find it, as you will be instinctively drawn to the crystals that will benefit you the most.

It is important to cleanse crystals prior to their use since they can absorb negative as well as positive energies. There are many methods but one of the most common methods is to cleanse them with water. Take them down to the sea, a stream or any source of fresh water or use bottled spring water. Allow your crystals to dry in the sun to energize them.

There are numerous ways of using crystals. You may wear them, carry them around in your pocket, place them onto your body, under your pillow, place them in a room or meditate with them.

The following are just a few of the many crystals that can assist detoxification not only of the spirit but the body and mind too.

- Amber – a marvellous stone for detoxification. Amber cleanses the body, mind and spirit and is thought to draw disease out of the body. It bestows joy and confidence and has an affinity for the kidneys, as well as the solar plexus and throat chakras.
- Amethyst – encourages a deep meditative state and is often worn as a stone of protection since it has the ability to clear negativity. An amethyst cluster is an excellent addition to a room. It helps to activate spiritual awareness.
- Aventurine – cleanses and protects the heart centre and encourages peace and harmony.
- Bloodstone (heliotrope) – purifies the chakras and clears away toxins from all the systems of the body.
- Carnelian – cleanses and balances the sacral chakra thus stimulating sexuality and creativity. Carnelian dispels negative emotions and protects and uplifts the spirit. It can even be used to cleanse other crystals.
- Chrysoprase – a vibrant apple-green crystal that eliminates waste from body, mind and spirit. It has an affinity for the

heart chakra, helping to mend a broken heart and transmuting jealousy, grief, envy and greed into positive emotions.

- Citrine (yellow quartz) – citrine is unusual in that it never needs to be cleansed. It clears the aura, filling any dark areas with light. Citrine is also an excellent energy booster.
- Fluorite – an excellent stone for purification of body, mind and spirit and also for rooms. Fluorite helps the mind to focus in meditation and opens up the intuition.
- Hematite – draws out negativity from the base chakra making us feel safe and secure. It also prevents you from absorbing any negativity from those around you.
- Lapis lazuli – thought by the ancient Egyptians to be a stone from heaven. Lapis heightens our intuition, promotes purification and provides protection.
- Malachite – a detoxifying stone for cleansing the body, mind and spirit. It encourages old traumas and past experiences to come to the surface to be released so that we can move on.
- Obsidian – detoxifies the chakras as well as purifies the body and mind. It cleanses a negative atmosphere, provides a protective shield and makes us feel secure and balanced. The Mayan priests used it for scrying to look into the future.
- Quartz – known as the 'master healer', quartz clears blockages from all the chakras and purifies negative energy. Wear or carry a piece of clear quartz to protect yourself from negativity and keep a piece at home and at work too!
- Tiger's eye – renowned for its ability to ward off the evil eye it is highly recommended for protection and for releasing toxins.
- Turquoise – detoxifies and balances all the chakras. Turquoise is often worn or carried to protect the wearer against negative influences and is a stone of balance.

Your mind and spirit detox summary

- Say at least one affirmation daily.
- Meditate for a few minutes daily.
- Practise the chakra cleansing exercise once a week (optional).
- Choose at least one Bach flower remedy for your detox.
- Select one essential oil to detox your mind and one to detox your spirit.
- Choose one crystal to cleanse your mind and spirit.

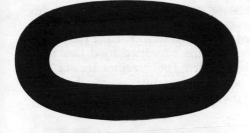

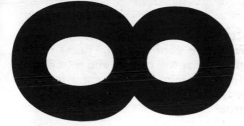

08

the detox recipes

In this chapter you will learn:
- about how to combine the permitted foods to create delicious meals.

The 21-day detox plan does not mean that you will have to starve yourself for three weeks. In this chapter you will find a whole host of delicious, tried and tested recipes. Each recipe, of course, includes only foods from the permitted food lists and does not break any of the detox rules. These recipes are not 'set in stone', so feel free to be as imaginative as possible and experiment and create your own dishes.

Juices

There is no better way to start the day than with a freshly made fruit, vegetable or fruit/vegetable combination. Juices are powerful nutritional supplements that will cleanse and revitalize you. Who needs a strong cup of coffee to get them going in the morning when you can have the energy boost of juices without the slump in energy afterwards?

Pineapple pep-you-up

Ingredients
2 slices pineapple
½ cucumber
1 apple, seeded

Directions
Feed the pineapple into the juicer followed by the apple and cucumber. Pour into a glass and serve immediately.

Apples are marvellous cleansers. They detoxify the liver and colon. As a source of pectin apples are useful for removing heavy metals from the body. Apples contain quercetin as well as other antioxidants and therefore help to protect against cancer, heart disease and premature ageing.

Pineapples also cleanse the liver and bowels. They aid digestion and combat sinus congestion. Pineapples, as well as apples and cucumber are a source of potassium which helps to regulate blood pressure. Cucumber cleanses the liver, bowels and kidneys and is excellent for reducing water retention.

Watermelon wake-up call

Ingredients
¼ watermelon, cut into pieces
1 orange, peeled (leave white pithy part)
A handful of seedless red/black grapes

Directions
Feed all the ingredients into the juicer, pour into a glass and drink immediately.

Watermelon is an excellent gentle diuretic. It provides potassium that helps regulate blood pressure and is an excellent source of beta-carotene and other antioxidants which mop up the free radicals preventing heart disease, cancer and premature ageing. Red and black grapes are a wonderful source of bioflavonoids and cleanse the liver, bowels, kidneys and lymphatic system.

Ginger zinger

Ingredients
3 carrots, tops removed
1 apple, seeded
25 mm (1 inch) fresh ginger root

Directions
Feed all the ingredients into the juicer, pour into a glass and drink immediately.

Both apples and carrots are very cleansing. Carrots detox the liver and colon and are a rich source of beta-carotene. The pectin in apples clears the heavy metals from the system and the quercetin is a powerful antioxidant.

Ginger is one of the best spices for improving the digestion. It is a well-known remedy for nausea, constipation, diarrhoea, wind and spasmodic pain. It is also excellent for boosting the circulation and really wakes you up!

Energy booster

Ingredients
Small handful of parsley
Small handful of watercress
Handful of spinach
2 carrots
1 apple, seeded

Directions
Juice all the ingredients together, pour into a glass and drink immediately.

Watercress, parsley and spinach are excellent sources of folic acid (as are all dark leafy-green vegetables), supply iron which helps to prevent anaemia and they give you a real energy boost. All the organs of elimination are cleansed. Carrots and apples are an excellent addition to any juice both for their therapeutic properties and their taste.

Berry reviver

Ingredients
1 cup raspberries
6 strawberries
1 cup of cherries, pitted
1 lime

Directions
Juice all the ingredients together, pour into a glass and drink immediately.

This juice is full of antioxidants, vitamin C and potassium. It will help eliminate toxins, boost the immune system and is an excellent tonic for the liver. You will feel refreshed and revitalized.

Other delicious combinations include:

- Apple, grape and ginger
- Carrot, apple and celery
- Blackcurrant, grape and apple
- Grapefruit and apple
- Tomato, cucumber and celery
- Orange, grape and melon
- Spinach, carrot, apple and alfalfa sprouts
- Carrot, apple, beetroot and ginger.

These are just a few of my personal favourites but please experiment with your own combinations. Remember that you can use any of the herbs and spices on the list to give your juices that extra special touch – cayenne, ginger and garlic are ideal. Herbs such as parsley and mint make great garnishes too! I have never had a disaster with fruit juices or fruit and vegetable juice combinations. However, green vegetable juices can be an acquired taste.

Smoothies

If you do not own a juicer but want to enjoy the benefits of fresh fruit then why not try making smoothies? They are packed full of vitamins and minerals. All you need is a food processor or blender. Bananas make particularly delicious smoothies. But make sure that your bananas are ripe – never green. If you ever find that you have too many ripe bananas then peel them and pop them into the freezer. Eat them raw for a delicious treat!

Always remove thick peel and stones and chop your chosen fruit into thick chunks or slices. Yoghurt or milk is sometimes added to a smoothie but remember this is a non-dairy detox so why not try soya milk, rice milk, oat milk, soya yoghurt, goats' milk yoghurt or sheep's milk yoghurt?

Frozen berries are often used in smoothies to make them cold. Some blenders will crush ice, in which case you could blend your ice cubes first followed by your fruit. Alternatively you could make your smoothies and serve in glasses with ice cubes.

To make your smoothies even more nutritious add a small handful of nuts or seeds. Almonds, cashews, sunflower, sesame or pumpkin seeds are particularly delicious!

Berry reviver smoothie

Ingredients
2 bananas, peeled and sliced
10–12 hulled strawberries (hulling strawberries removes their green caps and inner white cores)
1 cup raspberries
1 cup blueberries
1–2 cups cranberry juice

Directions
Put all the ingredients into a blender or food processor and blend until smooth.

Tropical island paradise smoothie

Ingredients
2 bananas, peeled and sliced
2 slices of fresh pineapple, cut into chunks
½ mango, peeled, stone removed, and chopped
1 kiwi, skinned
10–12 hulled strawberries
1–2 cups cranberry juice

Directions
Put all the ingredients into a blender or food processor and blend until smooth.

Fruit delight smoothie

Ingredients
2 nectarines, pips removed, and chopped
4 apricots
1 cup raspberries
Small carton soya yoghurt

Directions
Put the above ingredients into a blender or food processor and blend until smooth and creamy.

Banana and strawberry sensation

2 bananas, peeled and sliced
10–12 hulled strawberries
1 cup soya milk or rice milk

Directions
Place all the ingredients into a blender or food processor and process until fully blended.

Vitamin C packed smoothie

Ingredients
2 bananas, peeled and sliced
1 orange, peeled and segmented
2 kiwis, skinned
10–12 hulled strawberries
½ cup blueberries, blackberries or blackcurrants
1 cup orange juice

Directions
Place all the ingredients into a blender or food processor and process until smooth.

Perfectly peachy smoothie

Ingredients
2 bananas, peeled and sliced
2 peaches, stones removed
1 cup apple juice

Directions
Blend all the ingredients together using your blender or food processor until smooth.

Queen melon quencher smoothie

Ingredients
1 ripe melon
10–12 hulled strawberries

Directions
Cut the melon in half and de-seed. Scoop out the flesh and blend with the strawberries until smooth and creamy.

King of the jungle smoothie

1 banana, peeled and sliced
1 orange, peeled and segmented
½ mango, peeled, stone removed, and chopped
½ papaya, peeled and chopped
1–2 cups orange juice

Directions

Put all the ingredients into your blender or food processor and process until smooth.

Nourishing nectar smoothie

1 banana, peeled and sliced
1 nectarine, stone removed, and chopped
2 passion fruits
1–2 cups orange juice

Directions

Place all the ingredients into a blender or food processor and blend until smooth.

Hot date smoothie

Ingredients

2 bananas, peeled and sliced
6 dates, pitted
1 cup soya milk or rice milk

Directions

Blend all the ingredients together in your blender/food processor until smooth and creamy.

Breakfasts

Fresh fruit breakfast salad

Instead of a fruit juice or smoothie why not mix together your favourite fresh fruits and serve with soya yoghurt, goats' yoghurt or sheep's yoghurt?

If you desire, sprinkle a teaspoon of sesame seeds, pumpkin seeds or sunflower seeds over the top of the yoghurt.

For a more substantial breakfast:

Basic porridge

Ingredients
500 ml spring water
1 cup organic grade porridge oats
1 tbsp oatmeal

Directions
Bring the water to the boil in a saucepan. Stir in the porridge and oatmeal and cook at just under the boiling point for approximately 4–5 minutes, stirring frequently. The porridge will start to thicken so you will know when it is cooked.

Pour the mixture into bowls and add fresh fruit (bananas are particularly nourishing) or dried fruit such as raisins, cranberries or apricots and nuts and seeds according to your preference. You may trickle a teaspoon of honey on top although if you have added fruit it will be sweet enough.

Porridge is also delicious when sprinkled with cinnamon or nutmeg.

Why not try other grains such as buckwheat, millet or quinoa?

Basic museli

Ingredients
½ cup rolled oats
½ cup millet flakes
½ cup rye flakes
½ cup hazelnuts
1 handful raisins
1 handful pumpkin seeds
1 handful sesame seeds
1 handful sunflower seeds
1 cup dried fruit (banana, figs, pear, apple or apricots)

Directions
Mix all the above ingredients together and store in an airtight container. To this basic muesli add a cup of mixed dried fruit. Choose from dried banana, figs, pear, apple, apricots, etc.

Serve with soya milk, goats' milk, almond milk, oat milk or rice milk. Alternatively serve with any fruit juice or non-dairy yoghurt. Fresh fruits of your choice may be added to your basic muesli base.

Soups

A freshly made nutritious homemade soup is always far superior to any canned product. Soups can be made quickly as well as cheaply. A soup can be served at lunchtime, at the beginning of a meal or it can even be a main course in itself. Soups are an excellent way of ensuring that you eat all these healthy vegetables! These soups will serve up to four people depending on your appetite and whether you are serving them as a starter or main course.

Yellow split pea soup

Ingredients
2 cups of dried yellow split peas, washed and soaked in water overnight
5 or 6 cups of water
1 large onion, chopped
3 carrots, chopped small
1 small turnip cut into small cubes
Herbs to taste (see page 67)

Directions
Place the split peas in a large saucepan and cover well with water. Bring to the boil, reduce to a simmer and cook for about 1 hour or until the peas are soft and mushy. Add the chopped onion, carrots and turnip and cook for a further 20 minutes until everything is tender.

Tomato and lentil soup

Ingredients
1 ½ cups water
½ cup red or brown lentils
3 sticks celery, sliced
2 carrots, sliced
1 small onion, coarsely chopped

3 cloves garlic, crushed
Herbs to taste (see page 67)
3 tomatoes diced

Directions

In a large pot, bring the water to a boil. Add lentils, celery, carrots, onion, garlic and herbs. Reduce heat, and simmer for about 30 minutes until lentils are soft and mushy. Add the tomatoes and simmer until heated through for a further 5 minutes. You may need to add more water occasionally.

Cauliflower soup

Ingredients

1 large onion
1 cup cauliflower florets
2 carrots
2 leaves spinach
Herbs to taste (see page 67)

Directions

Add all the vegetables and herbs to the saucepan. Add enough water to just cover the vegetables in the pan. Bring to the boil and continue boiling for about 15 minutes until all are very tender. Drain, reserving the water. Put the vegetables in a blender and blend until smooth adding more cooking water as needed for desired consistency.

Broccoli soup

Ingredients

1 medium onion
Stick of celery
1–2 cloves garlic
1 cup broccoli florets
1 tbsp yeast extract, vegemite or an organic low-salt vegetable stock cube
1 tbsp lemon juice
Herbs to taste (see page 67)
Water

Directions

Sauté the onions, celery and garlic in a little olive oil. Add the stock and chopped broccoli (including stems). Add enough water to just cover the vegetables in the pan. Bring to the boil and continue boiling for about 15 minutes until the vegetables are tender. Stir in lemon juice. Purée in batches in the blender. Return to pan and heat through, but do not boil. Stir frequently. Serve hot or cold.

Try sautéing in some ginger (approx 25 g, 1 oz) for a really tasty broccoli and ginger soup!

Creamy potato and celery soup

Ingredients
1 tbsp extra virgin olive oil
2 sticks of celery, chopped
1 medium onion, chopped
750 g (1 lb 10 oz) potatoes, diced
1 tbsp yeast extract, vegemite or an organic low-salt vegetable stock cube
Herbs to taste (see page 67)

Directions
Heat the oil in a deep saucepan. Add the celery and onion and cook over a medium heat until tender. Add your potatoes and cook for 5 minutes, stirring occasionally. Add enough water to only cover the vegetables in the pan, yeast extract and herbs and bring to the boil.

Reduce to simmer and leave to cook with lid on for 20–30 minutes until the potato softens.

Let the mixture cool and mix in a blender until creamy.

Bean sprout soup

Ingredients
2 cups bean sprouts
5 cups water
1 clove garlic, peeled and minced
1 tbsp finely chopped Spanish or red onion
2 tbsp extra virgin olive oil

Directions

Wash the bean sprouts thoroughly in cold water. Place them in a medium-sized pan. Add the water, cover the pan and boil for about 25 minutes. Reduce heat to simmer. Add the minced garlic, chopped onion, and olive oil. Bring to the boil and simmer again for about 10 more minutes. Serve with cooked brown rice.

Salads

A salad makes an excellent healthy lunch and can be taken to work in an airtight container. It can also be served at the beginning of a meal as a first course.

There are probably millions of salad possibilities but the main ingredient of any salad is lettuce. For years the iceberg lettuce dominated the choice in salads but they are actually the least nutritious. As a general rule, the darker green the leaves, the more nutritious the salad green. For example, romaine or watercress have seven to eight times as much beta-carotene, and two to four times the calcium, and twice the amount of potassium as iceberg lettuce. By varying the greens in your salads, you can enhance the nutritional content as well as vary the tastes and textures. I suggest trying several kinds, such as romaine, red and/or green leaf, chicory, escarole, etc.

Why not try spritzing some extra virgin olive oil onto Romaine leaves and grill until slightly soft – these make an excellent hors d'oeuvre!

Salads are dependent upon the freshness and the quality of the raw ingredients. If you can buy organic produce or grow your own then so much the better! Remember to use your imagination when making a salad – add nuts such as cashews and pine nuts as well as seeds such as sesame, sunflower and pumpkin and even sprouted beans and seeds such as alfalfa, mung, lentil and chickpeas for variation and nutrition.

Overleaf are a few salad recipes which will serve four people:

Classic mixed salad

Ingredients
4–6 leaves assorted lettuce, torn or chopped
1 tomato, sliced or 10 cherry tomatoes
½ cucumber, sliced
½ grated carrot
5–6 radishes, sliced
3–4 mushrooms, sliced

Directions
Mix all the ingredients together in a large bowl and serve with the vinaigrette or lemon juice dressing (see page 162).

Energizing salad

Ingredients
2–3 leaves romaine, torn or chopped
2–3 leaves of leaf lettuce, torn or chopped
Several sprigs watercress
½ carrot, sliced
¼ cucumber, sliced
¼ cup walnuts, chopped
¼ cup sunflower seeds

Directions
Place all the ingredients into a large bowl, mix together and serve with the vinaigrette (see page 162) or your favourite dressing.

Carrot salad

Ingredients
1 large carrot, finely grated
1 tbsp finely chopped Spanish or red onion
2 tbsp lemon or lime juice
¼ cup raisins

Directions
Mix together in a large bowl and keep in the refrigerator until required.

Bean sprout salad

Ingredients

1 red pepper
1 small head romaine lettuce
1 small head leaf lettuce
2 cups bean sprouts
½ cup cucumber, diced
1 avocado, cubed
¼ cup cider vinegar
1 tsp extra virgin olive oil

Directions

Prepare the red pepper by washing, cut in half and remove seeds and membranes, then cut into small strips. Wash the lettuce, spin or blot dry and place in a plastic bag with a paper towel; seal the bag and refrigerate.

In a saucepan, bring 1 litre water to the boil. Add the bean sprouts and blanch for 2 minutes. Remove and run under cold water briefly. Immerse in a bowl of ice water for 1 minute, drain well. (Alternatively you can gently fry your bean sprouts in olive oil.)

In a large bowl, combine bean sprouts, diced cucumber, strips of red pepper and avocado cubes. Add the cider vinegar and olive oil to the bean sprout mixture and toss to combine (add 1 teaspoon of sesame oil if desired). Cover bowl tightly and refrigerate for 1 hour.

To serve, tear lettuce into bite-sized pieces and divide equally among 4–6 salad plates. Top with the sprout mixture. This salad needs no further dressing to be a delicious and healthy dish.

If you have sprouted your own beans or seeds you may add them to this salad.

Orange salad

Fruit and salad provide a lovely combination of flavours and colours. This makes a wonderful first course as a dinner party dish.

Ingredients

2 oranges, seeded and segmented
1 pink grapefruit, peeled and segmented
⅓ cup olive oil
Freshly ground black pepper
4–6 assorted lettuce leaves
1 tbsp walnuts
1 tbsp hazelnuts

Directions

Place your orange and grapefruit segments into a bowl and pour over the olive oil. Add the black pepper, mix thoroughly and chill.

Serve on lettuce leaves with the hazelnuts and walnuts sprinkled on top.

Other delicious combinations which can be served with or without salad leaves include:

- Apple, avocado, raisins and hazelnuts
- Melon, raisins, watercress and sunflower seeds
- Pineapple, avocado and pine nuts
- Apple, banana and walnuts.

Favourite dressings

Apple juice vinaigrette

Ingredients

4 tbsp extra virgin olive oil
2 tbsp organic cider vinegar
½ cup apple juice
½ teaspoon minced garlic (cut in tiny pieces)

Directions

Put all the ingredients in a screw top jar and shake well. Keep in the refrigerator and shake before serving.

You may wish to add some chopped herbs too!

Lemon juice dressing

Ingredients

6 tbsp extra virgin olive oil
2 tbsp freshly squeezed lemon juice
1 clove freshly crushed garlic
Freshly ground black/cayenne pepper

Directions

Place all the ingredients into a screw top jar and shake well. Store in the refrigerator and shake vigorously before serving. If you really cannot bear garlic (in spite of all its therapeutic properties) then add a few freshly chopped chives.

Hummus

Ingredients

1 can (400 g, 14 oz) of cooked chickpeas, drained
2 tbsp oil
2–3 cloves fresh garlic
2 tbsp light tahini (sesame paste)
1 lemon, freshly squeezed
Some water to blend
50 ml ginger water (steep some ginger in boiling water for about 10 minutes) (optional)

Directions

Place all the ingredients in a food processor and blend until fairly smooth.

By adding the ginger water the hummus will be more suitable as a dip for vegetables, or as a salad dressing. It is also excellent served with rice and vegetable dishes.

Store in a sealed jar in the refrigerator.

Avocado or guacamole dip

Ingredients

2 avocados, peeled and stones removed
1 small onion, finely chopped
2 cloves garlic, minced (use a garlic press for stronger flavour)
Juice of 1 lemon
Juice of 1 lime
¼ tsp cayenne pepper
(For guacamole) add 2 ripe diced tomatoes

Directions

Place all the ingredients in a food processor and blend or mash with a fork for a chunkier texture.

Main courses

All these recipes will serve at least four people.

Risotto

1 tbsp extra virgin olive oil
1 medium onion, peeled and chopped
½ litre water
1 tbsp yeast extract, vegemite or an organic low-salt vegetable stock cube
Herbs to taste (see page 67)
225 g (8 oz) cooked brown rice
50 g (2 oz) soya mince (cooked with liquid retained)
½ cup sweetcorn
½ red pepper, de-seeded and coarsely chopped
½ green pepper, de-seeded and coarsely chopped
6 large cabbage leaves
2 carrots (scraped and grated)

Directions

Pour the oil in a pan and cook the onion until golden brown. Add the water, stock, herbs and cooked soya mince and cook for five more minutes. Stir in sweetcorn, peppers and rice, cover and simmer for about 15 minutes or until the liquid has been reduced. In a pan of boiling water cook the cabbage leaves for about 5 minutes.

Arrange the cabbage leaves on a dish and pour the soya mixture into the centre, garnish with grated carrots and serve immediately.

Ratatouille

Ingredients
1 tbsp extra virgin olive oil
1 onion
1 red pepper, ½ green pepper
1 aubergine
1 clove garlic
2 x 400 g (14 oz) cans chopped tomatoes
Herbs to taste (see page 67)

Directions
Heat the oil in a saucepan. Chop the onion and fry for 1 minute. Roughly chop the peppers and aubergine, add to the pan and fry for another minute. Crush the garlic and add to the pan with the tomatoes and herbs. Bring to the boil, put the lid on the pan and simmer for 30 minutes, stirring occasionally. Take the lid off the pan, add a little water if necessary and stir well and simmer for 15 more minutes.

NB This recipe goes well with rice and hummus.

Try adding a sprinkling of cayenne pepper.

Rice-stuffed red peppers

Ingredients
3 red peppers
2 tbsp extra virgin olive oil + 1 tsp for brushing
1 onion, chopped
½ celery stick, sliced
¼ cup sliced mushrooms
30 g (1 oz) feta cheese
¼ cup chopped nuts (see page 64)
1½ cups cooked brown rice
Herbs to taste (see page 67)

Directions

Preheat the oven to 375°F, 190°C, gas mark 5.

Roast the peppers for approximately 20 minutes or until they start to singe. Remove from the oven and allow to cool. Slice off the tops of the peppers, remove the seeds and core (trim, chop and keep the tops for the next stage).

Heat the oil in a frying pan and sauté the onion until golden brown. Add the chopped pieces of red pepper, celery and mushrooms and continue to cook for a further 5 minutes. Add small pieces of feta cheese, chopped nuts, brown rice and herbs and mix thoroughly.

Fill the peppers with the mixture and brush each pepper with some olive oil then stand them in an oiled baking dish in a little water. Bake at 350°F, 190°c, gas mark 4 for 30 minutes until they brown or the filling melts.

Meatless lentil bolognese

1 litre water
250 g (9 oz) red or green lentils
2 tbsp extra virgin olive oil
1 onion, chopped
2 cloves garlic crushed
1 celery stick, sliced
2 x 400 g (14 oz) cans chopped tomatoes
Herbs to taste (see page 67)
1 carrot, scraped and grated

Bring the water to the boil, stir in the lentils and remove any scum from the surface. Cover and simmer for about 30 minutes or until the lentils are soft and mushy.

Heat the olive oil in a saucepan and add the onion, garlic and celery, stir frying until soft. Add the tomatoes and herbs, cover and simmer for 5 minutes. Pour in the lentils and cook for a further 5 minutes. Serve with a garnish of grated carrots.

Meatless shepherd's pie

Ingredients
175 g (6 oz) soya mince
¼ cup chopped nuts (see page 64)
4 potatoes
2 small onions (chopped)
2 leeks
1 clove garlic
3 carrots, scraped and grated
2 tbsp extra virgin olive oil
Herbs to taste (see page 67)

Directions
Heat the oven to 350° F, 177°C, gas mark 4. Cook the soya mince as instructed on the packet, adding the chopped nuts. Dice the potatoes and boil for 20–5 minutes until they are cooked but still firm, take them out and mash them. While you are waiting for the potatoes, slice the onions, leeks and garlic and, with the carrots, add to a pan and fry until soft in the olive oil.

Stir the cooked vegetables, soya mince mixture and herbs into an oiled lasagne-sized baking pan. Top with the mashed potatoes, smoothing them out at the top and bake in the oven for 30–40 minutes. Garnish suggestions: paprika, minced parsley, sesame seeds.

Vegetable and red kidney bean stew

Ingredients
1 tbsp extra virgin olive oil
2 large onions, sliced
2 leeks, sliced
1 red pepper, de-seeded and chopped
3 carrots, sliced
2 sticks celery, sliced
1 x 400 g (14 oz) can organic red kidney beans, rinsed and drained
or
125 g (4.5 oz) red kidney beans, soaked, rinsed and drained
4 tomatoes, chopped
½ tsp cayenne pepper

Directions

In a large saucepan heat up the oil and add the onions, leeks, pepper, carrots and celery. Place the lid on the pan and cook over a gentle heat for 15 minutes. Add the red kidney beans, tomatoes and cayenne. Cover and cook for 15–20 minutes and then serve with jacket potatoes or on a bed of steamed kale.

NB Why not try experimenting with other beans? Aduki beans and mung beans would go particularly well with this recipe.

Spicy vegetable casserole

Ingredients

2–3 tbsp extra virgin olive oil
2 onions, sliced
1 large clove garlic
1 tsp cardamom
1 tsp ground coriander
1 tsp turmeric
½ tsp cayenne
1 bay leaf
4 carrots, sliced
2 leeks, sliced
450 g (1 lb) potatoes, peeled and cut into cubes
150 ml water

Directions

In a large ovenproof casserole dish heat up the oil and fry the onions until soft. Stir in the garlic, spices and bay leaf. Then add the carrots, leeks and potatoes and stir them so that they are coated with the spices and olive oil. Now add the water and bring to a gentle boil. Cover and place in a warm oven (325°F, 163°C, gas mark 3) and bake for approximately 1½ hours or until tender.

Serve on a bed of brown rice.

Vegetable and bean casserole

Ingredients

1 tbsp olive oil
2 medium onions, chopped
2 litres water
3 carrots, diced

3 courgettes/zucchini, diced
1 cup cabbage, finely chopped
1 cup cauliflower florets
1 cup white kidney beans (cannellini); use either pre-cooked or organic canned beans
3 cloves garlic, crushed
Herbs to taste (see page 67 for options)
3 tbsp tomato purée
1 tbsp yeast extract, vegemite or an organic low-salt vegetable stock cube
1 tsp cayenne pepper
1 tsp cider vinegar

Directions

In a large pot and on high heat, fry the onions in the oil. After they are light brown put them in the water. Add all the other vegetables, including the garlic and herbs. After everything is boiling in the pan, cover and turn the heat down to simmer.

After all the vegetables are soft, add the tomato purée, then the yeast extract, cayenne pepper and the cider vinegar. Simmer everything for at least 3 hours allowing the flavours to permeate.

You may need to add more water occasionally due to the long cooking time.

Try experimenting with different seasonal vegetables.

Sole with ginger and lemon

Ingredients

4 sole fillets
1 dessertspoon extra virgin olive oil
½ onion, finely chopped
1 small piece of fresh ginger root
1 lemon

Directions

Although I have used sole you can choose any white fish fillet for this recipe. Preheat the oven to 350°F, 176°C, gas mark 4. Brush an ovenproof dish with a little extra virgin olive oil and place your sole fillets in it. Sprinkle your finely chopped onion over the fish and then grate fresh ginger all over the fillets. Squeeze the juice of the lemon liberally over the fish, cover loosely with foil and bake for approximately 20 minutes.

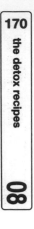

This dish is best served with a selection of fresh steamed vegetables or a crisp green salad.

Salmon and dill

Ingredients
4 salmon steaks
1 dessertspoon extra virgin olive oil
1 tbsp freshly squeezed lemon juice
2 tbsp fresh dill
cayenne pepper

Directions
Brush the salmon steaks with olive oil and grill until pink and tender. Combine the lemon juice and dill with any remaining olive oil, mixing well, and brush this dressing onto each salmon steak. Sprinkle with cayenne pepper.

Serve this dish with a fresh, crisp salad.

Fish in tomato sauce

Ingredients
2 tbsp extra virgin olive oil
1 onion, finely chopped
1 clove garlic, finely chopped
2 cups ripe tomatoes, chopped
1 tbsp parsley
½ tsp oregano
½ tsp thyme
450 g (1 lb) boneless white fish (e.g. cod/halibut), cut into pieces

Directions
Heat the oil in a saucepan and sauté the onion and garlic until tender and transparent in appearance. Add the chopped tomatoes, parsley, oregano and thyme. Bring up to a boil and gently simmer for 10–15 minutes, according to taste. Add the fish to the herby tomato sauce and simmer for approximately 5 minutes until the fish is tender.

Serve on a bed of brown rice.

Grilled tuna steaks

Ingredients
4 tuna steaks
2 tbsp extra virgin olive oil
Juice of a freshly squeezed lemon
1 clove garlic, crushed
Freshly ground black pepper

Directions
Arrange the tuna steaks in a shallow ovenproof dish. Combine the olive oil, lemon juice and crushed garlic in a small bowl. Pour this marinade over the tuna steaks and place in the fridge for 2 hours, turning from time to time. Grill the fish until tender and serve sprinkled with freshly ground black pepper.

This dish may be served with fresh vegetables or salad.

Desserts

Even though you are on a detox you can still have a dessert. Although many people eat fruit at the end of a meal they should really be eating it prior to a meal. Fruits are easily digested and should be eaten on an empty stomach. The best time to eat fruit is first thing in the morning which is why I recommend starting your day with fruit, fruit juices or smoothies. If you eat fruit after a meal unfortunately the food that you have eaten is still digesting. Any fruit that you eat now will have nowhere to go and will ferment. This will cause problems such as indigestion, flatulence and bloating.

Yoghurt

Directions
A pot of soya, goats' or sheep's yoghurt with a small teaspoon of honey drizzled in makes the perfect end to a meal. Sprinkle a handful of nuts or seeds of your choice over the yoghurt and honey for extra nutrition.

Cheese and celery platter

Directions
Place a selection of any goats' or sheep's cheese such as chèvre or feta on a plate. Add sticks of celery and red and green grapes. A simple yet delicious dessert.

Brown rice pudding

Ingredients

100 g (3.5 oz) brown rice
1 litre soya, almond, oat, rice or goats' milk
Pinch of nutmeg

Directions

Stir together the brown rice and milk in a casserole dish. Sprinkle a pinch of nutmeg into your mixture and bake uncovered on a low heat (300°F, 150°C, gas mark 2) for 2½–3 hours. Make sure that you stir your rice pudding a few times for the first 2 hours and then allow your pudding to become brown and crispy.

Serve each bowl with a teaspoon of honey and grated almonds if desired.

Sesame-rice cookies

Ingredients

1 cup sesame tahini
½ cup honey
A few drops vanilla extract
A few drops almond extract
½ cup chopped sunflower seeds, ground seeds or nuts
1 cup brown rice flour
1 tsp non-aluminium baking powder

Directions

Cream the tahini, honey, vanilla and almond extract together, then mix in the ground or chopped nuts or seeds.

Mix the rice flour and the baking powder together. Add to the sesame mixture.

Form into eight large balls and place on lightly oiled baking sheet. Flatten the balls slightly. Bake at 350°F, 177°C, gas mark 4 for 15–20 minutes or until barely golden.

These cookies have an excellent flavour, similar to peanut butter cookies.

taking it further

Fasting

Fasting is an ancient health remedy advocated by both Plato and the Egyptians. It is mentioned in the Bible throughout the book of Exodus and Jesus. Moses and Elijah all fasted for up to 40 days. Nowadays, Christians fast during Lent, Hindus often fast and Muslims fast during Ramadan.

Fasting is a rest from food that encourages our body's natural self-healing capacities. Fasting provides us with an opportunity for the elimination of toxins and rejuvenation. When a person is sick their systems are filled with poisons from the diet such as artificial colourings, flavourings and preservatives, pollutants, medications and many other toxins. Fasting enables a sick body to cleanse and heal. A whole host of ailments may improve with fasting such as allergies, skin diseases, digestive disorders, obesity, headaches, insomnia and arterial sclerosis. In addition, mental problems such as lack of clarity, nervousness, anger and frustration may be treated.

Fasting is also a way of preventing health problems from occurring. It also brings about weight loss and is even thought to extend life as shown by a research project in mice who were fasted every third day. Their life span increased by 40 per cent.

When should I fast?

An ideal time to fast is when not too many physical, emotional or mental stresses and strains are being put upon you. The perfect situation would be on a vacation to a warm country, although unfortunately most of us associate our holidays with the over consumption of food and alcohol!

If you do not want to use vacation time for fasting then choose any time of the year but avoid celebration times such as Christmas and birthdays as well as stressful periods. Probably the most important factor for a fast is your desire and enthusiasm to succeed. Do it when you feel the time is right!

Should everyone fast?

The 21-day detox plan that I have outlined is suitable for everyone except those individuals as detailed on page 32. I would not recommend fasting to anyone who has a very toxic diet. After following my detox plan, however, fasting would be an excellent idea.

There are many different types and lengths of fasts and I would never recommend anyone fasting for longer than two or three days without medical supervision.

Tips for fasting

- Never fast for more than three days without medical supervision.
- Always build up to your fast properly. At least three days of healthy eating (follow the rules of my detox plan) should precede any fast.
- Drink at least 2 litres of water per day whilst you are fasting – one glass of water per hour is a good guide. This will ensure that the toxins that are released are flushed out properly.
- Always pick a time when you know you can rest if you have too. You may feel tired and headachy during the fast and it is much better to lie down than to take painkillers.
- Never do any strenuous physical activity when fasting as it is a common side effect to feel light headed.
- During a fast your body temperature may well drop so be prepared with some warm clothing.
- Always break your fast properly. Eat fruit and vegetables – not egg, bacon and fried bread.

If you feel ready to give your body a spring clean then why not go for it? The first fast is the most difficult – regular fasters can carry on quite normally with their everyday activities. After a fast expect to feel uplifted, rejuvenated and energized. Your skin will glow and your eyes will be bright and shiny.

The one-day fruit fast

For maximum benefit chose any one fruit – apples, pears and grapes are particularly cleansing. Eat as much of your chosen fruit as you like throughout the day. Make sure that you drink your 2 litres of fluid in the form of water and/or juice, which should be the juice of your chosen fruit.

The one-day juice fast

You can drink as much organic fruit juice (preferably freshly made) as you want to. Once again only chose one fruit juice for best results.

The one-day water fast

On this fast you will only be drinking water. Drink one glass of water every hour throughout the day. I would recommend doing a fruit fast or a fruit juice fast prior to a water fast.

Fasting really is an excellent way of eliminating toxins. I would thoroughly recommend a one-day fast every month.

Useful addresses

Denise Brown Essential Oils Ltd
Kingshott Business Centre, 23 Hinton Road, Bournemouth, BH1 2EF
Tel: +44 (0)1202 708887
www.denisebrown.co.uk

Suppliers of special detox packs, skin brushes, Epsom salts, flower remedies and a wide selection of high quality pure unadulterated essential oils, base oils, creams and lotions.

Wholistic Research Company Ltd
Unit 1, Enterprise Park, Claggy Road, Kimpton, Hertfordshire,
SG4 8HP
Tel: +44 (0)1438 833100
www.wholisticresearch.com

Suppliers of high quality juicers, sprouting/wheatgrass products,
water purifiers, etc.

Herbs of Grace Ltd
20 Merlin Park, Fred Dennatt Way, Mildenhall, IP28 7RD
Tel: +44 (0)1638 712123/715715
www.herbsofgrace.co.uk

Provides flexible, balanced and effective herbal preparations.

Biocare Ltd
Lakeside, 180 Lifford Lane, Kings Norton, Birmingham, B30 3NU
Tel: +44 (0)121 433 3727
www.biocare.co.uk

Vitamin and mineral supplements, probiotics, herbal extracts
and nutriceutical combinations.

Higher Nature
The Nutrition Centre, Burwash Common, TN19 7LX
Tel: +44 (0)1435 884668
www.higher-nature.co.uk

Vitamin and mineral supplements.

Great Smokies Diagnostic Laboratory/Genovations™
63 Zillicoa Street, Asheville, NC 28801, USA
Tel: +1(828) 253 0621

Comprehensive digestive stool analysis.

Beaumont College of Natural Medicine
http://www.beaumontcollege.co.uk

Information on professional training courses under the direction
of Denise Whichello Brown.

index